# VITAMINS
# & MINERALS:
## The Health Connection

Health Plus Enrichment Series

# VITAMINS & MINERALS:
## THE HEALTH CONNECTION

A Complete Fingertip Reference Book

by ANNI AIROLA LINES, R.D.

**Health Plus Publishers**

Phoenix, Arizona

# VITAMINS AND MINERALS
## The Health Connection

**Library of Congress Cataloging in Publication Data**

Lines, Anni M.
  Vitamins and minerals.

  (Health Plus enrichment series)
  Bibliography: p.
  Includes index.
  1. Vitamins in human nutrition--Handbooks, manuals,
etc. 2. Minerals in human nutrition--Handbooks, manuals,
etc. 3. Food--Vitamin content--Handbooks, manuals, etc.
4. Food--Mineral content--Handbooks, manuals, etc.
I. Title. II. Series [DNLM: 1. Minerals-popular works.
2. Nutrition--popular works. 3. Trace Elements--popular
works. 4. Vitamins--popular works. QU 160 L754v]
QP771.L55  1985         641.1'7         85-7638
ISBN 0-932090-14-1  (pbk.)

Published by
Health Plus Publishers
PO Box 22001, Phoenix, AZ 85028


Printed in the United States of America

# TABLE OF CONTENTS

# SECTION 2: MINERALS

# SECTION 3: VITAMIN & MINERAL PURCHASE & USE GUIDE

# SECTION 4: TABLES

# PUBLISHER'S PREFACE

As more people become aware that vitamins and minerals play a vital role in their health and well-being, it becomes increasingly important that they *understand the significance* of that role. Certainly vitamins and minerals are not new, however, and there have been other books written on the subject, so why publish another one?

For two very good reasons:

1. *Vitamins and Minerals: The Health Connection,* by Anni Airola Lines, R.D., offers concise "one-stop" information on *everything* you need to know about vitamins and minerals:

What is this vitamin (or mineral)?
What does it do?
How much do I need?
What are the best food sources?
When is supplementation advisable or necessary?
What happens if I don't get enough?
What happens if I get too much?

In addition to detailed information on each vitamin and mineral individually, there is a handy chart that tells at a glance the functions, deficiency symptoms, toxicity symptoms, food sources, Recommended Dietary Allowances, and complimentary nutrients of all the vitamins and minerals. There is an expanded table of the Best Food Sources of selected nutrients; there are tips for buying, storing, and taking food supplements and vitamins; there is a section on natural vs. synthetic vitamins and an easy way to help you determine which is which. In other words, this fully indexed and referenced book is the *COMPLETE* guide to minerals and vitamins in an easily readable and condensed, yet detailed, form.

We are confident that this book measures up to the standards of excellence that Health Plus Publishers has maintained throughout its twenty-year history. We are proud to present the first book in the Health Plus Enrichment Series, *Vitamins and Minerals: The Health Connection.*

— HEALTH PLUS PUBLISHERS

# INTRODUCTION

Vitamins and minerals, along with proteins, carbohydrates, and essential fatty acids, are required by every part of the body to maintain health and prevent disease. Vitamins and minerals referred to as "essential" are those which it is necessary to obtain through dietary intake in order for the body to function normally. A Recommended Dietary Allowance (RDA) or Estimated Safe and Adequate Intake has been established for these substances. Other vitamins, such as choline and para-aminobenzoic acid (PABA) of the B-complex, while necessary for the normal function of the body, are produced in sufficient quantities by the body; therefore there has been no need for dietary intake established for the healthy person. No essential nutrient function has ever been established for laetrile or pangamic acid, wrongly referred to as vitamins $B_{17}$ and $B_{15}$ respectively. Therefore, they are not included in this vitamin reference book.

Although each vitamin and mineral has specific functions within the body, many vitamins and minerals work together to help each organ function efficiently. This is the process of synergism, whereby two substances working in cooperation produce an effect which neither could produce alone, or which is greater than the total effect produced by each substance working alone. In addition to keeping you healthy, when taken in large amounts, vitamins and minerals can act as drugs to aid in the treatment of disease.

Ideally, all nutrients should be obtained from the foods you eat, but in today's fast-paced society, this is very difficult to do. Many people now consume convenience foods which are nutritionally inferior due to extensive processing, chemical additives, and lengthy storage. In addition, emotional and physical stress, weight-loss diets, illness, medications, etc., increase the need for many vitamins and minerals beyond that which can normally be obtained from foods.

Many studies show that Americans are not getting even the RDA of vitamins and minerals from their diets. Although actual deficiencies are rare in this country, subclinical deficiencies are more common than was once thought. For example, many children do not get enough vitamins A and C or calcium and iron, and women are often deficient in calcium and iron. Women past menopause have a greater need for calcium and vitamin D. Bear in mind also, that there is a gap between the amount of a nutrient necessary to prevent an *actual deficiency* and the amount needed to keep your body running at its *peak level of health.* Prolonged marginal supplies of essential nutrients will ultimately result in the devastation of vital cells and tissues, leading to vulnerability to disease, both acute and chronic. Most doctors and other health practitioners now recognize the need for vitamin supplementation on a regular basis to maintain good health. Vitamin and mineral deficiencies are best treated by small amounts; mega vitamin therapy, although currently popular, is not necessary for the treatment of most deficiencies or disease symptoms.

The purpose of this book is to provide a concise, yet complete, guide to understanding how vitamins and minerals function, to help you determine if you may need to supplement your diet, to help answer some basic questions, and to provide information on the best food sources for each vitamin and mineral. When considering food sources, we have eliminated most meats as well as processed foods and refined carbohydrates. Our lists have been compiled from the most healthful wholesome foods

— fresh fruits and vegetables, whole grains, nuts and seeds, dairy products, and seafoods. As you consider food sources of the various nutrients, be aware that even "fresh, wholesome foods" can become nutritionally inferior due to any number of factors such as depleted or polluted soil, improper storage and handling before they reach your kitchen, and improper preparation. Therefore, it becomes increasingly difficult to obtain *all* the vital nutrients through proper diet alone.

It is logical to assume that nearly everyone could benefit from the inclusion of vitamin and mineral supplements in their daily diet. For some people it means the difference between simply existing at a low level of well-being and optimum health; for others it means the difference between life and death. Self-diagnosis or self-treatment of illness should always be avoided however. No information presented in this book is intended to be, nor should it be interpreted to be, diagnostic or prescriptive. Before beginning any supplementation program, it is very important to consult a physician familiar with nutritional therapies and abide by his advice. A list of such practitioners is available from the International Academy of Biological Medicine, P.O. Box 31313, Phoenix, Arizona 85046. Please send a self-addressed, stamped envelope for your free copy.

# SECTION 1

# VITAMINS

## Understanding Vitamins

According to *Taber's Cyclopedic Medical Dictionary* (Clarence W. Taber, F. A. Davis Company, Philadelphia, PA, 9th ed.), vitamins are extremely complex organic (carbon-containing) substances essential in very small amounts to support normal growth and maintain health. They are not sources of energy, nor do they contribute in a significant amount to the substance of the body, but they *are* essential for normal metabolism and body functions. Some vitamins can be synthesized in the intestines by naturally-occurring bacteria, but most vitamins must be provided in the diet. A lack of essential vitamins will lead to various deficiency symptoms. Whole grains, nuts and seeds, dark green leafy vegetables, yellow vegetables, and fruits are the best food sources of most vitamins.

Vitamins function in the body in two major ways: (1) As components of enzyme systems (coenzymes) that function as catalysts, vitamins help to accelerate certain

7

chemical reactions essential for health. These enzymes help regulate the metabolism of proteins, carbohydrates, and fats, and participate in the formation of bones, tissues, blood cells, and hormones; and (2) Excess vitamins beyond what the body needs for normal growth and health maintenance may act as drugs or chemicals.

Vitamins are classified as either *fat soluble* or *water soluble*. The fat soluble vitamins — A, D, E, and K — need dietary fat or bile salts in order to be absorbed through the intestinal wall and stored in the body. Diseases that interfere with the digestion of fat, excessive intake of mineral oil, or lack of bile salts may prevent absorption of the fat soluble vitamins and lead to deficiencies. The fat soluble vitamins are stored in the body, so it is not necessary to consume them every day. In fact, too much may accumulate in the body and cause toxicity symptoms to develop. The best food sources of the fat soluble vitamins are whole grains, fish liver oils, and vegetables.

Water soluble vitamins in excess of immediate needs, however, are excreted in the urine and not stored in the body. They should, therefore, be provided in the diet on a daily basis. These vitamins — the B-complex and vitamin C — are also more easily destroyed by factors such as overprocessing, extreme heat and light, and improper preparation and storage.

The *Recommended Dietary Allowances* (RDA) of nutrients for healthy populations have been established by the Food and Nutrition Board of the National Research Council. The RDA are considered adequate to meet the nutritional needs of healthy persons involved in light physical activity and living in a moderate climate, and provide a reasonable margin of safety for each vitamin. However, there are many situations that may require adjustments in the amount of nutrients required by an individual, including increased physical activity, climate, aging, infections, disease, metabolic disorders, injuries, infections involving the gastrointestinal tract resulting in impaired absorption of nutrients, and differences in genetic makeup (biochemical individuality).

The RDA should be exceeded in cases of medically diagnosed deficiencies. These are rare, however, except among alcoholics, those with defects in intestinal absorption, the poor, the pregnant, and the elderly. Certain disease conditions are also treated with large doses of vitamins. Continued use of certain prescription drugs may increase the body's need for specific nutrients. Women taking oral contraceptives, for example, need extra $B_6$, riboflavin, folic acid, and vitamin C. Pregnant women need increased amounts of all vitamins. Stress may increase the need for vitamin C.

The nutritional needs of each person are different, and must be evaluated on an individual basis. Avoid self-diagnosis or self-treatment. Before considering a supplementation program, consult your physician. The deficiency symptoms described in this book occur only after a prolonged inadequate dietary intake or an inability of the body to absorb and metabolize nutrients. Similar symptoms could be caused by a variety of diseases or disorders, and may not be indicative of a vitamin deficiency. If symptoms are present in spite of an adequate intake of nutrients, consult a nutritionally and holistically oriented physician and abide by his advice.

# Part 1

# THE
# FAT SOLUBLE
# VITAMINS

# Vitamin A

Vitamin A, a fat soluble vitamin readily found in many foods, is one of the nutrients found to be inadequate in the typical American diet. The activity of vitamin A is measured as preformed vitamin A (retinol), found only in animal sources, and provitamin A carotenoids from plant sources. Butter and cream may contain both forms of vitamin A. The average diet contains half the total vitamin A activity as retinol and half as provitamin A carotenoids. Beta Carotene has the highest vitamin A activity and is the most plentiful of the carotenoids. These carotenes are active and useful to the body only after being converted into retinol (vitamin A) during or after absorption. The thyroid hormone, thyroxin, stimulates this conversion of carotene to vitamin A.

Vitamin A is measured as retinol equivalents. One retinol equivalent (RE) is equal to one microgram (mcg.) of retinol or six micrograms of Beta carotene. See table 1.

---

**Table 1**

| 1 I.U. Vitamin A | = 0.3 mcg. retinol |
|---|---|
| | 0.6 mcg. B-carotene |
| 1 retinol equivalent (RE) | = 1 mcg. retinol |
| | 6 mcg. B-carotene |
| | 12 mcg. other |
| | carotenoids |
| | 3.33 I.U. retinol |
| | 10 I.U. B-carotene |

---

The absorption and utilization of vitamin A may be decreased by gastrointestinal disorders such as ulcerative colitis, obstruction of the bile ducts, cirrhosis of the liver, infections, or excessive intake of iron, alcohol, and mineral oil. Diabetics may have an impaired ability to convert carotene to vitamin A.

Both vitamin A and carotene are stable in the presence of heat. With vitamin A, as with many other nutrients, interaction with other vitamins and minerals is important. Zinc is necessary for the utilization of vitamin A, and oxidation of vitamin A stored in the body may be prevented by vitamins C and E.

# RDA

Infants. . . . . . . . . . . . . . 400 - 420 mcg. RE (1300 I.U.)
Children . . . . . . . . 420 - 700 mcg. RE (1300 - 2300 I.U.)
Adult females . . . . . . . . . . . . 800 mcg. RE (2700 I.U.)
Adult males . . . . . . . . . . . . 1000 mcg. RE (3300 I.U.)

# Functions

- Increases resistance to infections, especially respiratory infections, by maintaining and repairing epithelial tissues — the mucous linings and membranes of the body and the skin.
- Speeds wound healing; useful in acne and other skin disorders.
- Helps prevent cancer of the epithelial tissues by maintaining healthy skin and mucous membranes.
- Extends youthfulness and prevents premature aging and senility by strengthening the tissues in the cell walls.
- Improves oxygenation of tissues by increasing the permeability of blood capillaries.

- Important in the secretion of gastric juices, in the metabolism of proteins, glycogen synthesis, formation of some hormones, and ribonucleic acid (RNA) production.
- Essential for the growth of cartilage, bones, and teeth in infants.
- Counteracts night blindness and weak eyesight by helping in the formation of visual purple (rhodopsin) in the rods of the retina, and visual violet in the cones of the retina for color vision.
- Promotes healthy eye tissues and may have some protective effect against glaucoma.
- Involved in the production of estrogen and androgens (sex hormones).
- Essential during pregnancy and lactation; may improve fertility and help prevent miscarriage.
- Helps maintain sperm levels and healthy testicular tissue.
- Helps counteract the harmful effects of a polluted environment on the mucous membranes.

## Deficiency Symptoms

Prolonged deficiency may result in:
- Increased susceptibility to infections, especially in the respiratory and urinary tracts.
- Night blindness (the eye takes longer to adjust from bright light to dim light).
- Itching and dryness of the eyes; damaged eye tissues (xerophthalmia) leading to blindness in young children.
- Retarded growth in children due to impaired metabolism.
- Loss of vitamin C.
- Lack of appetite, poor sense of taste and smell.

- Soft tooth enamel, periodontal disease.
- Rough, scaly, dry skin.
- Acne, boils, psoriasis, and premature wrinkles.
- Dry dull hair, dandruff, hair loss.
- Brittle, ridged fingernails which may peel.

# Toxic Effects

More than 15,000 RE (50,000 I.U.) taken daily over a long period of time can cause toxic symptoms:

- Loss of hair, dry skin and ulcerations; cracked lips.
- Joint and bone pain.
- Irritability, headache, fatigue; blurred vision.
- Loss of appetite, abdominal pain, nausea, vomiting, diarrhea.
- Interference with normal skeletal development in infants and young children.
- Transient hydrocephalus in infants.
- Excessive intake of carotene containing foods can cause yellowing of the skin.

# Natural Sources

- Fruits — mangos, cantaloupe, apricots, papayas.
- Vegetables — sweet potatoes, carrots, pumpkin, collard greens, sweet red peppers, spinach, dandelion greens, turnip greens, kale, winter squash, mustard greens, broccoli, Swiss chard, beet greens, tomatoes, asparagus.
- Dairy — eggs, butter, cheese, milk.
- Other — fish liver oils, liver.

The best food sources of vitamin A are fish liver oils, liver, yellow fruits and vegetables, green leafy vegetables, and dairy products.

(See Table 3 — BEST FOOD SOURCES OF SELECTED NUTRIENTS, page 131.)

# Vitamin D

Vitamin D, the "sunshine vitamin," is present in both animal and plant tissues. The two most important substances possessing vitamin D activity are $D_2$ (ergocalciferol) and $D_3$ (cholecalciferol). $D_2$ is produced synthetically by ultraviolet irradiation of the plant sterol, ergosterol. $D_3$ is the naturally occurring form of vitamin D in animal tissues. It is formed by the action of sunlight on 7-dehydrocholesterol in the skin. Both $D_2$ and $D_3$ appear to be equally effective. Vitamin D is measured as micrograms of cholecalciferol; 10 mcg. of cholecalciferol is equal to 400 I.U. of vitamin D.

Vitamin D is stable in foods, and is not adversely affected by storage, processing, or cooking. It is efficiently absorbed from the gastrointestinal tract unless there is malabsorption of fat due to a lack of bile salts, pancreatic insufficiency, or a defect in the function of the intestinal mucosa. Because vitamin D is stored in the body, it is potentially toxic in large doses. There appears to be no health benefits to healthy individuals if they take more than the RDA of vitamin D. Vitamin D is most effective when taken in combination with vitamin A.

## RDA

Infant and Children. . . . . . . . . . . . . . 10 mcg. (400 I.U.)
Adults . . . . . . . . . . . . . . . . 5 - 10 mcg. (200 - 400 I.U.)

## Functions

- Regulates calcium and phosphorus absorption and metabolism along with the parathyroid hormone,

thereby helping to maintain a positive calcium balance.
- Important in infancy and adolescence for the proper mineralization of bones and teeth.
- Prevents rickets.
- Helps prevent tooth decay and periodontal disease.

# Deficiency Symptoms

Prolonged deficiency may result in:
- Rickets, a childhood disease characterized by retarded growth, poor bone formation, and malformed teeth.
- Osteomalacia, a softening of the bones in adults, leading to shortening, fractures, and muscle spasms.
- Muscular weakness.
- Poor assimilation of minerals.
- Reduced parathyroid activity.

# Toxic Effects

- Anorexia; nausea; vomiting.
- Excessive thirst; excessive urination.
- Calcium may be withdrawn from the bones and deposited in soft tissues, resulting in calcification of the heart, kidneys, lungs, blood vessels, and skin.
- Kidney stones.
- Increased lead absorption.

# Natural Sources

- Vitamin D is produced by sunshine or ultraviolet light acting on oil normally present on the skin and is then absorbed through the skin. However, exposure to sunlight may be inadequate during winter months, or due to increased ozone in the atmosphere.

- Food sources include fish liver oils, egg yolks, fortified milk, butter, cheese, liver, tuna, salmon, shrimp, sardines, and mushrooms.

# Vitamin E

Vitamin E is made up of eight tocopherols and tocotrienols, d-alpha-tocopherol being the most active form. The tocopherols are natural antioxidants. They inhibit the oxidation of unsaturated fats, fat soluble vitamins, vitamin C, and the B-complex vitamins. The biological activity of vitamin E is measured as International Units (IU) or milligrams (mg.) One mg. of natural vitamin E as d-alpha-tocopherol is equal to 1.49 IU. Synthetic vitamin E is less potent, with one mg. of dl-alpha tocopherol being equal to 1.1 IU.

The requirement for vitamin E increases when large amounts of polyunsaturated fats or oils are included in the diet. Known antagonists (substances which interfere with or destroy vitamin E in the body) are inorganic iron, synthetic estrogen and chlorine or chlorinated water.

Vitamin E is stored in the body, but excess amounts are excreted in the urine. Therefore, this vitamin is considered relatively non-toxic. Since large amounts of vitamin E can increase blood pressure, however, those with heart disease, high blood pressure, or diabetes should not take this vitamin in large amounts. Begin with small doses under the direction of a physician.

## RDA

Infants . . . . . . . . . . . . . . . . 3 - 4 mg. ∝ TE* (4.5 - 6 IU)
Children. . . . . . . . . . . . . . 5 - 7 mg. ∝ TE (7.5 - 10.5 IU)
Adults . . . . . . . . . . . . . . . 8 - 10 mg. ∝ TE (12 - 15 IU)

*alpha-tocopherol equivalent

# Functions

- Makes more oxygen available to the tissues, thereby reducing the need for oxygen.
- As an antioxidant, helps to slow down aging by preventing the formation of free radicals.
- Improves circulation by dilating the blood vessels.
- Effective as an antithrombin and a natural anticoagulant.
- May increase the levels of high-density lipoprotein (HDL) and decrease the levels of low-density lipoprotein (LDL), LDL being the cholesterol responsible for clogging the arteries.
- By improving circulation and reducing clotting, vitamin E is effective in the prevention and treatment of heart disease, angina pectoris, thrombophlebitis, leg ulcers, "restless" legs, and varicose veins.
- Speeds healing of burns, cuts, abrasions, bedsores, and cold sores, and helps prevent scar formation.
- Eases the pain of cold sores and shingles.
- Helps protect the lungs and other tissues from damage by pollutants.
- Retards the aging process by preventing oxidation and acting as a detoxifying agent.
- Helps maintain cell membranes.
- Involved in the prevention and treatment of reproductive disorders, infertility, miscarriage, still births, menstrual and menopausal disorders.
- Also used in treatment of emphysema, asthma, arthritis, migraine headaches.

# Deficiency Symptoms

Prolonged deficiency may result in:
• Heart disease; pulmonary embolism; strokes.
• Degeneration of tissues in the testicles.
• Reproductive disorders; miscarriages; sterility.
• Muscular disorders; fatigue.
• Blurred vision.
• Increased fragility of red blood cells.

# Toxic Effects

Vitamin E is the least toxic of the fat soluble vitamins. Only 30-40% of the vitamin E ingested is absorbed, and very little is stored in the body. Excess vitamin E is eliminated from the body more quickly than the other fat soluble vitamins. Therefore, vitamin E is considered less likely to cause adverse effects than A or D.

Excessive levels of vitamin E may increase blood pressure and cause skin rashes, fatigue, and weakness. Those with high blood pressure, chronic rheumatic heart disease, or hyperthyroidism should avoid high does of vitamin E.

# Natural Sources

• Grains - oats, wheat, rye, barley, brown rice.
• Fruits - apples.
• Vegetables - green leafy vegetables, asparagus, cabbage, green peas, sweet potatoes.
• Dairy - eggs, butter, cheese.
• Nuts and seeds - raw or sprouted seeds.

- Other - Unrefined cold-pressed vegetable oils such as wheat germ oil, sunflower seed oil, or olive oil; fresh wheat germ (less than one week old - rancid wheat germ is not a good source of vitamin E); legumes.

The best food sources of vitamin E are vegetable oils.

(See Table 3 - BEST FOOD SOURCES OF SELECTED NUTRIENTS, page 132.)

# Vitamin K

Vitamin K, the "anti-hemorrhaging" or "coagulation" vitamin, is present in several forms. $K_1$ and $K_2$ are found in foods and can be manufactured by bacteria in the intestinal tract — approximately half the vitamin K used by the body is produced by normal intestinal flora. Vitamin $K_1$ (phylloquinone) is found in leafy green vegetables, while vitamin $K_2$ (menaquinone) is found in animals, and produced by bacteria. Several synthetic forms, including menadione and phytonadione have been produced.

Prolonged antibiotic therapy, excessive intake of mineral oil, diarrhea, ulcerative colitis, gall stones, liver disease, cancer, and kidney disease are among factors that may interfere with the production of vitamin K in the intestines, and with absorption of vitamin K from foods, thereby leading to a deficiency.

## RDA

Estimated Safe and Adequate Intake:

Infants . . . . . . . . . . . . . . . . . . . . . . . . . . . . 10 - 20 mcg.
Children . . . . . . . . . . . . . . . . . . . . . . . . . . . 15 - 60 mcg.
Adults  . . . . . . . . . . . . . . . . . . . . . . . . . . . 70 - 140 mcg.

## Function

- Necessary for the formation of prothrombin, which is required for blood clotting.
- Important for normal function of the liver.
- Vitality and longevity factor.

- Involved in the process of phosphorylation, whereby glucose is converted to glycogen.
- May be necessary for the maintenance of normal bone metabolism.

# Deficiency Symptoms

Prolonged deficiency may result in:
- Hemorrhages in the body (nosebleeds, bleeding ulcers, intestinal bleeding, blood in the urine or eye, postoperative bleeding, etc.) due to prolonged bloodclotting time.
- Miscarriage.

# Toxic Effects

- High doses of synthetic vitamin K may cause jaundice in infants due to an increased breakdown of red blood cells.
- No known toxicity to natural vitamin K, since very little is stored in the body.

# Natural Sources

- Vegetables - asparagus, cauliflower, watercress, turnip greens, broccoli, cabbage.
- Dairy - milk, egg yolks, cheese.
- Other - kelp, liver, blackstrap molasses, soybean oil, safflower oil, fish liver oil.

The best food sources of vitamin K are green leafy vegetables.

# Part 2

# THE
# WATER SOLUBLE
# VITAMINS

# Vitamin B₁
## (Thiamine)

Thiamine, known as the anti-beriberi, anti-neuritis, and anti-aging vitamin, is a component of the coenzyme thiamine pyrophosphate (TPP), which is necessary for the breakdown of carbohydrates. By this process, glucose is oxidized in the cells to produce energy.

Thiamine is stable in dry form, but is quickly destroyed when exposed to water, neutral or alkaline solutions, air, heat, or overcooking. It can be stored in an acid solution for some time before loss of activity. Freezing has very little adverse effect on thiamine.

Because it is a water soluble vitamin and is not stored in the body, thiamine must be present in the diet every day. Deficiencies can be induced by excessive alcohol and dietary sugars, and an excess of processed and refined foods. Thiamine can be destroyed by the enzyme thiaminase, which is present in raw sea food, and by chlorine from drinking water. Renal disease, chronic febrile infections, smoking, pregnancy, lactation, surgery, and oral contraceptives can increase the amount of thiamine used by the body. Tea and coffee contain a thiamine antagonist which may prevent the absorption and use of thiamine.

## RDA

Infants................................. 0.3 - 0.5 mg.
Children.............................. 0.7 - 1.2 mg.
Adults ................................ 1.0 - 1.5 mg.

# Functions

- Necessary for the breakdown of carbohydrates to produce energy.
- Promotes growth and repair of tissues.
- Indispensable for the health of the nervous system, heart, muscles, and intestines.
- Improves digestion and peristalsis and helps prevent constipation.
- Helpful in the prevention of fatigue and edema.
- Increases stamina and improves mental attitude.

# Deficiency Symptoms

Prolonged deficiency may result in:
- Loss of appetite; impaired hydrochloric acid production leading to digestive disorders; constipation; weight loss.
- Muscular weakness; irritability; loss of memory; mental depression; fatigue; insomnia.
- Heart irregularities; weak heart muscles.
- Beriberi, characterized by neuritis and edema.

# Toxic Effects

There is no known toxicity; however, some individuals may be sensitive to repeated injections of thiamine, resulting in irritability, insomnia, headache, weakness, and rapid pulse.

# Natural Sources

- Grains - millet, oats, buckwheat, rye, wheat.
- Vegetables - potatoes, turnip greens, collards, asparagus, bean sprouts, green peas.

- Dairy - milk, cheese, eggs.
- Nuts and seeds - nuts; all seeds, especially sunflower seeds.
- Other - brewer's yeast, torula yeast, legumes, liver.

The best food sources of thiamine (vitamin $B_1$) are whole grains, brewer's yeast, and nuts and seeds.

(See Table 3 - BEST FOOD SOURCES OF SELECTED NUTRIENTS, page 133.)

# Vitamin B₂
## (Riboflavin)

Riboflavin is a component of several flavoprotein enzyme systems which are necessary for normal cellular respiration. These enzyme systems work closely with other enzymes containing niacin and thiamine in reactions involving the release of energy from glucose and fatty acids formed from the breakdown of carbohydrates, fats, and proteins.

Like all the B vitamins, riboflavin is water soluble and fragile. The major losses in processing are due to leaching into water. Riboflavin is destroyed by light and strong alkaline solutions; however, it is relatively stable in the presence of heat, and it is resistant to oxidation. Since it is not stored in the body, riboflavin must be supplied in the diet regularly. Pregnancy, lactation, stress, oral contraceptives, excess consumption of processed and refined foods, and low calorie diets can increase the need for riboflavin.

## RDA

Infants.............................0.4 - 0.6 mg.
Children..........................0.8 - 1.4 mg.
Adults ............................1.2 - 1.7 mg.

## Functions

- Involved in the breakdown of carbohydrates, fats, and proteins to release energy.
- Essential for protein metabolism.

- Necessary for growth and wound healing, and during pregnancy and lactation.
- Helps maintain normal red blood cell count.
- Protects against damaging effects of pollutants and drugs.
- Important for the health of the eyes, skin, nails, and hair.
- May help prevent cataracts.
- Aids the cells in the utilization of oxygen.

# Deficiency Symptoms

Prolonged deficiency may result in:
- Increased sensitivity to light; bloodshot eyes; itching and burning of eyes; blurred vision; cataracts.
- Sore, burning red tongue; cracks on the lips and in the corners of the mouth.
- Loss of appetite; digestive disturbances; loss of weight.
- Dull, dry hair or oily hair; hair loss; split nails.
- Oily skin; eczema; dermatitis.
- Anxiety; fatigue; dizziness.
- Anemia.
- Vaginal itching.

# Toxic Effects

None known.

# Natural Sources

- Grains - all whole grains; millet, wheat germ, wheat bran.
- Fruit - avocados.

- Vegetables - green leafy vegetables, broccoli, asparagus, mushrooms, winter squash, yams.
- Dairy - milk, cheese, eggs.
- Nuts and seeds - almonds, sunflower seeds.
- Other - liver, torula yeast, brewer's yeast, soybeans.

The best sources of riboflavin (vitamin $B_2$) are liver, brewer's yeast, and dairy products.

(See Table 3 - BEST FOOD SOURCES OF SELECTED NUTRIENTS, page 134.)

# Vitamin $B_3$
## (Niacin)

The anti-pellagra vitamin, niacin (nicotinic acid), is converted to the active form nicotinic acid amide (niacinamide) in the body. Niacin is a component of two coenzyme systems — nicotinamide-adenine dinucleotide (NAD) and nicotinamide-adenine dinucleotide phosphate (NADP). These coenzymes play an important role in cell membrane metabolism in oxidation-reduction reactions vital to the use of carbohydrates, fats, and proteins as sources of energy.

The body can manufacture niacin from the amino acid tryptophan. It takes 60 milligrams of tryptophan to produce 1 niacin equivalent (NE) or 1 mg. of niacin. This conversion of tryptophan to niacin may be impaired by a deficiency of vitamin $B_6$. The need for niacin increases during pregnancy, lactation, illness, or periods of growth. Diets low in other B vitamins or protein, and high in refined sugars and starches will deplete the body of niacin.

Niacin is more resistant to destruction by air, light, heat, acids, alkalies, and long storage than are thiamine or riboflavin.

# RDA

| | |
|---|---|
| Infants | 6 - 8 mg. NE |
| Children | 9 - 16 mg. NE |
| Adults | 13 - 19 mg. NE |

# Functions

- Vital as a coenzyme in the breakdown of carbohydrates, fats, and proteins for energy sources.
- Dilates blood vessels and increases the flow of blood to peripheral capillaries, improving circulation and reducing high blood pressure.
- Reduces cholesterol and triglyceride levels.
- Helps maintain normal growth, healthy skin, and normal functions of the gastrointestinal tract and nervous system.
- May be effective in treating or preventing migraine headaches.
- Mega doses of niacin are used in the treatment of schizophrenia.
- Involved in the formation of many hormones, including thyroxine and insulin.
- Helps stimulate the production of hydrochloric acid and bile salts.

# Deficiency Symptoms

Prolonged deficiency may result in:
- Poor appetite; indigestion.
- Coated tongue; halitosis; canker sores.
- Muscular weakness; fatigue.
- Skin lesions.
- Irritability; nervousness; memory loss; insomnia.
- Chronic headaches; depression; mental dullness; disorientation.
- Severe prolonged deficiency may cause pellagra, which is characterized by dermatitis, diarrhea, dementia.

# Toxic Effects

Doses of 100 mg. or more of niacin (nicotinic acid) can cause the release of histamine, which aggravates asthma and peptic ulcers, and may have a side effect known as "flushing." This flushing, or burning and itching of the skin, is caused when the blood vessels dilate and blood rushes to the skin. It is considered harmless, and usually last for about 15 minutes. Some people enjoy this sensation. Nicotinic acid amide (niacinamide) does not cause this flushing reaction.

Although niacin is a water soluble vitamin, some of this vitamin is stored in the liver. Large amounts of niacin should not be taken in the presence of liver damage or gastrointestinal ulcers. Excess niacin may result in gouty arthritis, skin problems, cardiac arrythmias, and elevated plasma glucose levels.

# Natural Sources

- Grains - whole wheat, millet, brown rice, wheat germ, rice bran.
- Fruits - dates, dried fruits, mangos, cantaloupe, avocados, peaches.
- Vegetables - asparagus, mushrooms, corn, collards, winter squash, potatoes.
- Dairy - milk, cheese, eggs.
- Nuts and seeds - nuts, especially almonds; sunflower seeds, sesame seeds.
- Other - liver, fish, brewer's yeast, legumes, torula yeast.

The best food sources of niacin (vitamin $B_3$) are liver, whole grains, potatoes, and brewer's yeast.

(See Table 3 - BEST FOOD SOURCES OF SELECTED NUTRIENTS, page 135.)

# Vitamin B$_6$
## (Pyridoxine)

The vitamin B$_6$ group consists of pyridoxine, pyridoxal and pyridoxamine. Pyridoxine occurs mainly in plants; pyridoxal and pyridoxamine are found in animal products. All three forms are functionally interrelated and equally active.

Pyridoxal phosphate and pyridoxamine phosphate function as active coenzymes necessary for normal carbohydrate and protein metabolism. They are involved in transamination, which is the transfer of an amino group from an amino acid to other compounds to produce new, non-essential, amino acids in the body. The B$_6$ group also functions as a coenzyme for many other enzyme systems, and seems to work more efficiently in the presence of the other B-complex vitamins, magnesium, and vitamin C.

Pregnancy, lactation, stress, aging, and excess protein and sucrose increase the need for B$_6$. Gastrointestinal disorders and various drugs deplete the body of vitamin B$_6$. Estrogen in oral contraceptives increases the metabolism of tryptophan, which uses up B$_6$, and could lead to a deficiency. Choline, essential fatty acids, biotin, and pantothenic acid seem to decrease the need for B$_6$. Since cooking, processing, and storage destroy vitamin B$_6$, the best sources are fresh raw foods.

## RDA

| | |
|---|---|
| Infants | 0.3 - 0.6 mg. |
| Children | 0.9 - 1.6 mg. |
| Adults | 1.8 - 2.2 mg. |

# Functions

- Coenzyme involved in carbohydrate, protein, and fat metabolism.
- Involved in the formation of red blood cells, and in the production of antibodies which protect the body against bacterial infections.
- Helps control nausea and vomiting during pregnancy.
- May be effective in treating degenerative diseases, elevated cholesterol, some types of heart disease, and diabetes.
- Vitamin $B_6$ is required for the absorption of vitamin $B_{12}$ and for the production of hydrochloric acid.
- Helps maintain the health of the skeletal system and teeth.
- Improves skin disorders such as acne.
- As a natural diuretic, may relieve premenstrual edema.
- Regulates the balance between sodium and potassium in the cells.
- May prevent or reduce epileptic seizures.
- May relieve tingling, numbness, pain, and swelling in the hands due to carpal tunnel syndrome.

# Deficiency Symptoms

Prolonged deficiency may result in:
- Sore mouth, lips, and tongue; halitosis.
- Dermatitis; eczema; hair loss.
- Anemia; edema; increased infections; low blood sugar.
- Weakness; weight loss.
- Kidney stones; tooth decay.

- Depression; irritability; nervousness; confusion; apathy; insomnia; migraine headaches; convulsions.
- Tingling, numbness, pain and stiffness of joints; cramps in arms and legs.

# Toxic Effects

- Nervous system dysfunction.
- Seizures in infants whose mothers took excess vitamin $B_6$ during pregnancy.
- Interferes with L-dopa used to treat Parkinson's disease.

# Natural Sources

- Grains - brown rice, whole wheat, rye, oats, buckwheat, wheat germ, wheat bran.
- Fruits - bananas, cantaloupe, avocados, dried fruits, mangos.
- Vegetables - cabbage, broccoli, yams, potatoes, carrots, green peppers, green leafy vegetables, brussel sprouts, corn, cauliflower, green peas.
- Dairy - milk, cheese, egg yolks.
- Nuts and seeds - hazelnuts, walnuts, sunflower seeds, sesame seeds.
- Other - brewer's yeast, soybeans, garbanzos, peanuts, blackstrap molasses, liver, fish, such as salmon, mackerel, halibut, and tuna.

The best food sources of pyridoxine (vitamin $B_6$) are whole grains, bananas and other fruits, and seeds.

(See Table 3 - BEST FOOD SOURCES OF SELECTED NUTRIENTS, page 136.)

# Vitamin $B_{12}$

Vitamin $B_{12}$ is a group of cobalt-containing substances known as cobalamins. Because of its red crystalline form, vitamin $B_{12}$ is also known as the "red vitamin." The predominant forms of vitamin $B_{12}$ in animal tissues are methylcobalamin, adenosylcobalamin, and hydroxocobalamin. Cyanocobalamin is present in the body in very small amounts, but is the most stable form. It is the form produced by the fermentation of bacteria for commercial use.

In order to be absorbed, vitamin $B_{12}$ must be accompanied by an enzyme called the intrinsic factor. (If given in large doses, some vitamin $B_{12}$ will be absorbed without the presence of the intrinsic factor, however.) This factor is produced by glands in the stomach and is normally found in the gastric juice. The intrinsic factor combines with calcium to release $B_{12}$ into the intestinal mucosa.

Pregnancy, lactation, excessive protein in the diet, a strict vegetarian diet, alcohol, malabsorption syndromes, the use of laxatives, and aging will increase the need for vitamin $B_{12}$. Deficiencies of $B_6$, calcium, and iron may decrease the absorption of $B_{12}$, thereby increasing the need for dietary intake.

Vitamin $B_{12}$ is relatively stable in the presence of heat. Less than 30% of vitamin $B_{12}$ activity is lost during cooking.

## RDA

Infants. . . . . . . . . . . . . . . . . . . . . . . . . . . . 0.5 - 1.5 mcg.
Children. . . . . . . . . . . . . . . . . . . . . . . . . . 2.0 - 3.0 mcg.
Adults . . . . . . . . . . . . . . . . . . . . . . . . . . . . . 3.0 mcg.

# Functions

- Involved in the metabolism of carbohydrates, proteins, and fats.
- Important catalyst in the mitochondria of all cells.
- Plays a role in nucleic acid metabolism and the formation of RNA and DNA.
- Essential for the production of red blood cells, thereby helping to prevent anemia.
- Promotes absorption of iron, as well as the absorption of carotene and its conversion to vitamin A.

# Deficiency Symptoms

Prolonged deficiency may result in:

- Pernicious anemia — caused by a lack of intrinsic factor in the gastric secretions which prevents vitamin $B_{12}$ from being absorbed.
- Poor appetite; weakness; weight loss; chronic fatigue.
- Retarded growth in children.
- Loss of memory; depression; mood changes; difficulty in concentrating.
- Numbness; stiffness; difficulty in walking; loss of balance; prickly sensation in the skin.

# Toxic Effects

None known.

# Natural Sources

- Grains - oats, wheat germ.
- Dairy - milk, eggs, cheese, whey.

- Nuts and seeds - sunflower seeds.
- Other - liver, oysters, fortified brewer's yeast, spirulina, kelp, pollen, soybeans, peanuts.

The best food sources of vitamin $B_{12}$ are liver and dairy products.

Because $B_{12}$ is present in plant foods in such small amounts, vegetarians who do not use dairy products should supplement their diets with brewer's yeast or vitamin $B_{12}$ tablets. Fermented foods can supply some $B_{12}$, and very small amounts of this vitamin are produced by bacteria in the nodules of plant roots.

(See Table 3 - BEST FOOD SOURCES OF SELECTED NUTRIENTS, page 137.)

# Biotin

Biotin is a water soluble, sulfur containing member of the B-complex vitamins which is found in small amounts in all animals and plants. Biotin is normally produced by bacteria in the intestines. This bacterial synthesis may be inhibited by antibiotics, and/or a lack of riboflavin, niacin, and pantothenic acid in the diet.

Because biotin is found in so many foods, deficiencies are rare; however, a deficiency of biotin can occur if large amounts of raw egg whites are consumed. Avidin, a protein in the egg white, binds with biotin in the intestines, where it is synthesized, and prevents it from being absorbed. Cooking inactivates the avidin.

## RDA

Estimated Safe and Adequate Intake:
Infants . . . . . . . . . . . . . . . . . . . . . . . . . . . . . 35 - 50 mcg.
Children . . . . . . . . . . . . . . . . . . . . . . . . . 65 - 120 mcg.
Adults . . . . . . . . . . . . . . . . . . . . . . . . . 100 - 200 mcg.

## Functions

- Involved as a coenzyme in the metabolism of carbohydrates, proteins, and fats.
- Important in the metabolism of folic acid and vitamin $B_{12}$.
- Aids in the synthesis of ascorbic acid.
- May help prevent hair loss and improve growth and health of the hair.

# Deficiency Symptoms

Prolonged deficiency may result in:
* Loss of appetite; nausea; pallor; anemia.
* Eczema; seborrhea; dandruff; hair loss.
* Fatigue; confusion; depression.
* Muscle pain; heart abnormalities.
* Impairment of fat metabolism; high cholesterol levels.

# Toxic Effects

None known.

# Natural Sources

* Grains - brown rice, whole wheat, buckwheat, oats, barley.
* Fruits - most fruits, including berries, cherries, grapes, currants, cantaloupe, peaches, grapefruit, bananas, apples, avocados.
* Vegetables - asparagus, beet greens, carrots, mushrooms, spinach, tomatoes, corn, lima beans, cauliflower, onions, peas.
* Dairy - milk, cheese, egg yolks.
* Nuts and seeds - walnuts, almonds.
* Other - liver, brewer's yeast, kidneys, fish, blackstrap molasses, peanuts, soybeans.

The best natural sources of biotin are liver, egg yolks, nuts, and vegetables.

(See Table 3 - BEST FOOD SOURCES OF SELECTED NUTRIENTS, page 138.)

# Choline

Choline, a part of the B-complex, is widely distributed in most plants and animals. It is also manufactured by the body when adequate amounts of vitamin $B_{12}$, folic acid, and methlonlne (an amino acid) are available.

According to the latest revision of the *Recommended Dietary Allowances,* the average diet contains 400-900 mg/day of choline. No RDA have been established for choline since it is not considered essential for man. Deficiency symptoms have been observed in animals, but not in humans.

## RDA

Not established

## Functions

- Choline works with inositol as a part of lecithin (phosphatidylcholine) where it is involved in the transport of fat soluble substances, including the fat soluble vitamins A, D, E, and K.
- Necessary for the manufacture of sphingmyelin, a phospholipid essential for the health of the nervous system.
- Important as a precursor of acetylcholine which is essential for the transmission of nerve impulses.
- Helps reduce deposits of fats and cholesterol in the liver and arteries.
- Necessary in the synthesis of the nucleic acids, DNA and RNA.

- Helps prevent the formation of gallstones and improves liver and gallbladder function.
- Used in the treatment of nephritis, atherosclerosis, high blood pressure, glaucoma, and cirrhosis of the liver.

# Deficiency Symptoms

Prolonged deficiency may lead to:
- Cirrhosis and fatty infiltration of the liver.
- High blood pressure; atherosclerosis; arteriosclerosis.

# Toxic Effects

None known.

# Natural Sources

- Grains - whole grains, wheat germ.
- Vegetables - green leafy vegetables.
- Dairy - egg yolks.
- Other - granular or liquid lecithin from soybeans, liver, brewer's yeast, fish, legumes.

The best food sources of choline are lecithin, egg yolks, and liver.

# Folic Acid

Folic acid (pteroylglutamic acid), also known as folate or folacin, is a member of the B-complex vitamins. Folic acid coenzymes work closely with vitamin C and $B_{12}$. Although it is a water soluble vitamin, some folic acid is stored in the liver. It is rapidly destroyed by heat and light. Overcooking can destroy as much as 80% of the folic acid present in food.

Pregnancy, lactation, stress, aging, illness, and the use of alcohol, antibiotics, estrogen, or oral contraceptives may increase the need for folic acid. An iron deficiency may affect the metabolism of folic acid, particularly in pregnant women, thereby necessitating increased dietary intake. Folic acid, vitamin $B_6$, $B_2$ (riboflavin), and vitamin $B_{12}$ are all required together for the normal metabolism of protein.

Folic acid and vitamin $B_{12}$ are important in the treatment of nutritional macrocytic anemia and sprue. Pernicious anemia of pregnancy due to a poor diet and increased fetal demands is also treated with folic acid. Megaloblastic anemia in infants is due to folic acid and ascorbic acid deficiency; megaloblastic anemia in adults may be due to a deficiency of folic acid and ascorbic acid, or vitamin $B_{12}$. Indiscriminate use of folic acid supplements can hide a deficiency of vitamin $B_{12}$.

## RDA

Infants . . . . . . . . . . . . . . . . . . . . . . . . . . . . 30 - 45 mcg.
Children . . . . . . . . . . . . . . . . . . . . . . . . . 100 - 300 mcg.
Adults . . . . . . . . . . . . . . . . . . . . . . . . . . . . . . 400 mcg.

# functions

- Folic acid coenzymes are important as catalysts in the transfer of single carbon units to form amino acids.
- Necessary for the metabolism of protein with vitamin C and $B_{12}$ and the formation of RNA and DNA.
- Involved in hemoglobin metabolism and the formation of red blood cells.
- Involved in the synthesis of choline.
- May help prevent premature graying of the hair.
- Necessary for the maintenance of a normal pregnancy and for the prevention of congenital abnormalities.
- Works with hormones such as estrogen, testosterone, and the growth hormone, STH.
- Used in the treatment of atherosclerosis, circulation problems, stomach ulcers, menstrual problems, radiation burns and injuries, and infections.
- Important in the treatment of sprue, a nutritional deficiency disease characterized by anemia and acute diarrhea.

# Deficiency Symptoms

Prolonged deficiency may result in:
- Nutritional macrocytic anemia; megaloblastic anemia; and pernicious anemia of pregnancy.
- Glossitis (inflammation of the tongue); inflamed gums.
- Loss of hair; graying of hair; gray-brown skin pigmentation.
- Impaired absorption of all nutrients.
- Diarrhea; sprue; poor growth.

- Muscular weakness; fatigue; dizziness; depression; headaches.
- Spontaneous abortion; difficult labor; post-partum hemorrhaging; high infant mortality rate; birth defects.
- Poor circulation.

## Toxic Effects
None known.

## Natural Sources
- Grains - whole wheat, oatmeal, wheat germ.
- Fruits - cantaloupe, berries, oranges, bananas, avocados.
- Vegetables - brussels sprouts, beets, asparagus, green beans, lettuce, potatoes, mushrooms, carrots, broccoli, spinach.
- Dairy - milk, cheese, eggs.
- Nuts and seeds - nuts, sesame seeds.
- Other - liver, brewer's yeast, legumes.

The best food sources of folic acid are leafy green vegetables, fruits, dairy products, liver, and wheat germ.

(See Table 3 - BEST FOOD SOURCES OF SELECTED NUTRIENTS, page 139.)

# Inositol

Inositol, a part of the B-complex, is present in large amounts in the heart, brain, spinal cord, nerves, and cerebrospinal fluid. It is synthesized by the body within the cells. In plants and grains, inositol occurs as phytic acid, which binds calcium and iron and interferes with their absorption. Inositol is present in animal sources as phospholipid. It is estimated that 1 gram/day is consumed in the average American diet. Seven percent of the inositol ingested is converted to glucose. Diabetics excrete large amounts of inositol in the urine. Caffeine may deplete the body's supply of inositol.

## RDA

Not established.

## Functions

- Works with choline as a part of lecithin; involved in fat metabolism.
- Helps prevent hardening of the arteries and reduces blood cholesterol.
- Necessary for healthy heart, liver, and kidneys.
- May help prevent hair loss.
- May be useful in the treatment of obesity and schizophrenia.

## Deficiency Symptoms

Prolonged deficiency may lead to:
- Constipation.
- Eye abnormalities.

- High blood cholesterol and heart disease.
- Hair loss; eczema; dermatitis.

# Toxic Effects

None known.

# Natural Sources

- Grains - wheat germ, oatmeal, wheat, corn.
- Fruits - citrus, cantaloupe.
- Vegetables - green peppers, tomatoes, potatoes, zucchini.
- Dairy - milk.
- Nuts and Seeds - nuts.
- Other - liver, brewer's yeast, lecithin, legumes.

The best sources of inositol are liver and whole grains.

# Pantothenic Acid

As a part of the B-complex, pantothenic acid is widely distributed in foods, making deficiencies unlikely. It can be synthesized by bacteria in the intestinal tract, but is destroyed by exposure to heat, acids, and alkali. Pantothenic acid improves the function of the adrenal cortex by increasing the production of cortisone and other adrenal hormones. In the latest edition of the *Recommended Dietary Allowances,* the average intake in the United States was estimated at 7 mg. per day, with a range of 5 20 mg. per day.

## RDA

Estimated Safe and Adequate Intake:

| | |
|---|---|
| Infants | 2 - 3 mg. |
| Children | 3 - 5 mg. |
| Adults | 4 - 7 mg. |

## Functions

- Pantothenic acid (pantothenate) is a part of a catalyst called co-enzyme A (co-acetylase) which is involved in the release of energy from carbohydrates, proteins, and fats.
- Improves the production of cortisone and other hormones of the adrenal glands.
- As an anti-stress factor helps the body withstand physical and mental stress.
- Increases resistance to infections by aiding in the formation of antibodies.
- May help counteract damage caused by excessive radiation.

- Involved in the synthesis of cholesterol, steroids, and fatty acids.

# Deficiency Symptoms

Prolonged deficiency may lead to:
- Chronic fatigue; decreased resistance to infections; dizziness; muscular weakness.
- Stomach distress and constipation.
- Mental depression; irritability; insomnia.
- Graying and loss of hair.
- Skin diseases.
- Adrenal exhaustion; retarded growth.
- Low blood pressure.
- Muscle cramps; painful and burning feet.
- May contribute to allergies and asthma.

# Toxic Effects

None known.

# Natural Sources

- Grains — buckwheat, brown rice, oats, rye, wheat, wheat germ, wheat bran.
- Fruits — pomegranates, papayas, berries, figs, cantaloupe, oranges, mangos, dates, avocados, currants.
- Vegetables — green vegetables, corn, broccoli, sweet potatoes, mushrooms, kale, cabbage, cauliflower, asparagus, pumpkin, green peas.
- Dairy — milk, cheese, whey, eggs.
- Nuts and seeds — walnuts, cashews, almonds, pecans, sunflower seeds.
- Other — liver, brewer's yeast, legumes.

The best food sources of pantothenic acid are liver, eggs, whole grains, vegetables, and fruits.

(See Table 3 — BEST FOOD SOURCES OF SELECTED NUTRIENTS, PAGE 140.)

# Para-aminobenzoic Acid
## (Paba)

Para-aminobenzoic acid (PABA) is a part of the B-complex which has not as yet been determined to be necessary for humans. PABA is produced by bacteria in the intestinal tract. These bacteria may be destroyed by sulfa drugs, thereby contributing to a deficiency of PABA.

## RDA
Not established.

## Functions
- Involved in the production of folic acid.
- Involved in the formation of red blood cells.
- Along with pantothenic acid, choline, and folic acid, may be useful in preventing gray hair.
- May be helpful in treating eczema, lupus erythematosis, burns, and sunburn.
- In an ointment may protect the skin against sunburn and help prevent skin cancer and skin changes due to aging.

## Deficiency Symptoms
Prolonged deficiency may result in:
- Extreme fatigue; irritability; depression.
- Anemia.
- Eczema; gray hair; vitiligo.
- Reproductive disorders; infertility; loss of libido.

# Toxic Effects

High doses may cause nausea and vomiting.

# Natural Sources

- Grains — whole grains, wheat germ, bran.
- Vegetables — mushrooms.
- Dairy — milk, eggs, yogurt.
- Nuts and seeds — sunflower seeds.
- Other — liver, brewer's yeast, molasses.

The best food sources of PABA are liver and whole grains.

# Vitamin C

Vitamin C (ascorbic acid) is a water soluble vitamin easily destroyed by heat, light, and oxygen and the use of copper and iron cooking utensils. The requirements for vitamin C are increased during pregnancy and lactation, by infections, surgery, burns, injuries, stress, aging, smoking and the use of oral contraceptives. Vitamin C should be taken in several small daily doses rather than in one large dose because the excess vitamin C is rapidly excreted in the urine. It will be more effectively utilized if the supply is more equally distributed.

## RDA

Infants.................................35 mg.
Children ..............................45 mg.
Adults.................................60 mg.

## Functions

- Essential for the synthesis and health of collagen, the "intercellular cement."
- Strengthens all connective tissues, skin, bones, teeth, joints, muscles, tendons, cartilage, and capillaries.
- Protects vitamins A and E, and the B-complex vitamins — thiamine, riboflavin, pantothenic acid and folic acid — from oxidation.
- Essential for the formation of the adrenal and thyroid hormones.
- As a natural antihistamine, vitamin C helps reduce the symptoms of the common cold and allergies.

- Helps prevent the development of infected, bleeding gums in periodontal disease.
- May help in the treatment of urinary tract infections by inhibiting the growth of bacteria in the urine.
- May help lower cholesterol levels in the blood.
- Interferes with the conversion of nitrates and nitrites to nitrosamines and nitrosamides, known carcinogens.
- Improves absorption of iron from foods.
- Involved in converting folinic acid to folacin.
- Helps protect against toxic chemicals in the environment: cadmium, lead, mercury, ozone, carbon monoxide, PCB's, vinyl chloride, nitrates, nitrites, various drugs, etc.
- Promotes healing of wounds, burns, and bacterial infections.
- Helps the body deal with physical and mental stress.

## Deficiency Symptoms

Prolonged deficiency may result in:
- Tooth decay; periodontal disease.
- Slow healing of fractures and wounds.
- Lowered resistance to infections.
- Inability of the body to handle toxic effects of drugs and environmental pollutants.
- Severe deficiency causes scurvy, a disease that is eventually fatal. Scurvy results in a deterioration of collagen and capillary weakness and hemorrhaging. Symptoms of scurvy include: weakness; fatigue; shortness of breath; swollen, spongy, bleeding gums; loose teeth; hemorrhage in joints and skin; aching bones, joints, and muscles; osteoporosis; compressed vertebrae; rough, dry brown skin.

# Toxic Effects

Vitamin C is relatively non-toxic in large doses (1 gram/day or more) because it is rapidly excreted in the urine. Some symptoms may occur, however with megadoses (2 gram/day or more):

- Skin rashes; diarrhea.
- Excessive urination; irritation of the urinary tract; kidney stones.
- False positive tests for glucosuria.
- Vitamin $B_{12}$ deficiency.
- Withdrawal symptoms (scurvy) when high doses are suddenly discontinued.

# Natural Sources

The best sources of vitamin C are fruits and vegetables as listed below:

- Fruits — papayas, guavas, citrus fruits, cantaloupe, strawberries, rosehips, black currants, acerola cherries, persimmons, mangos.
- Vegetables — red and green peppers, parsley, broccoli, brussels sprouts, turnip greens, kohlrabi, collards, kale, cauliflower, potatoes, tomatoes, cabbage, asparagus.

(See Table 3 — BEST FOOD SOURCES OF SELECTED NUTRIENTS, page 141.)

# Bioflavonoids

Citrin, hesperidin, rutin, flavones, and flavonals are water soluble components of the bioflavonoids, or vitamin P. They are found in foods as part of the vitamin C complex and have a synergistic effect on vitamin C. No RDA have been established for the bioflavonoids. Rutin is derived from buckwheat leaves. Excess amounts of bioflavonoids are excreted through the urine and perspiration.

## RDA

Not established.

## Functions

- Strengthen capillary walls and help prevent hemorrhaging in the capillaries and connective tissues.
- Prevent vitamin C from being destroyed by oxidation.
- Enhance the absorption and utilization of vitamin C.
- Important in cases of respiratory infections, varicose veins, hemorrhaging, bleeding gums, eczema, hemorrhoids, radiation sickness, hypertension, coronary thrombosis, arteriosclerosis.

## Deficiency Symptoms

Prolonged deficiency may result in:
- Capillary fragility.
- Diminished vitamin C activity.
- Susceptibility to hemorrhages and bruising.

# Toxic Effects

None known.

# Natural Sources

- Grains — buckwheat.
- Fruits — citrus fruits, especially the pulp; grapes, apricots, strawberries, black currants, cherries, prunes, rosehips.
- Vegetables — fresh vegetables, especially green peppers.

The best sources of bioflavonoids are fruits and vegetables.

# SECTION 2

# MINERALS

## Understanding Minerals

Minerals are inorganic substances (containing no carbon) which play a vital role in the human body. They are essential components of respiratory pigments, enzymes, and enzyme systems; they regulate the permeability of cell membranes and capillaries. They function in the regulation of the excitability of muscular and nervous tissue. They are necessary for the regulation of osmotic pressure equilibria. They are essential for maintenance of a proper acid-alkaline balance; they are necessary constituents of glandular secretions, and they play an important role in water metabolism and regulation of blood volume. *(Taber's Cyclopedic Medical Dictionary)*.

The major, or *macrominerals*, make up 4% of the total body weight, and include calcium, phosphorus, magnesium, potassium, sulfur, chloride, and sodium. They function primarily as constituents of bones, teeth, muscles, blood, and nerve cells, and as soluble salts which help maintain the fluid balance and the acid-base balance within the body.

69

The *microminerals,* or trace elements, are present in the body in minute amounts and are usually involved as components of coenzymes and hormones to regulate body functions. They make up only 0.01% of total body weight. The most important trace elements are iron, zinc, iodine, copper, manganese, fluoride, chromium, selenium, and molybdenum.

Bromide, cadmium, vanadium, tin, nickel, aluminum, silicon, and cobalt are trace elements that are present in the body in minute quantities, and which have not been found as yet to be essential. Very little is known about their functions in the body. Deficiency symptoms of these micronutrients have not been observed.

All minerals work together in a delicate balance. Mineral salts and water are excreted daily from the body, and must be replaced through dietary intake. Minerals in excess of what is required for good health, however, are stored in the body and can build up to toxic levels if taken when not needed, or in large amounts. An excess of one mineral may then interfere with the function of other minerals. An insufficient supply of minerals can also upset the balance. The optimum diet should provide all the essential minerals in the proper balance for good health.

When considering therapeutic supplementation with minerals, as with vitamins, it is essential to consult a nutritionally oriented physician to avoid toxicity and mineral imbalances through improper supplementation.

Supplements in their natural forms, such as sea water, mined minerals, mineral water, kelp, and the natural foods mentioned in this book are the best choices for ensuring that your body is receiving all the minerals and trace elements it needs. For detailed information on therapeutic uses of vitamins and minerals, see *How To Get Well,* by Dr. Paavo O. Airola.

# Part 1

# THE
# MACROMINERALS

# Calcium

Calcium, the mineral Americans are most likely to be deficient in, is the most abundant mineral in the body, making up 2% of the total body weight. Ninety-eight percent of the calcium is found in the bones, 1% in the teeth, and 1% in the soft tissues. Calcium is constantly moving in and out of the bones, 1/5 of the calcium in the bones being replaced each year.

Adequate amounts of vitamins A, D, and C, as well as hydrochloric acid are necessary for the efficient absorption of calcium and phosphorus. Phosphorus and magnesium are required for calcium to be effective. Vitamin D, working with the parathyroid hormone, helps to maintain a constant level of calcium in the blood.

The need for calcium increases during pregnancy, lactation, growth during childhood and adolescence, emotional stress, and menopause, when low estrogen levels reduce calcium absorption. Inactivity, lack of exercise, excessive stress, high protein intake, and high fluoride intake may increase the amount of calcium excreted.

Only 30% of the calcium in the diet is absorbed. Some substances found in foods are known to interfere with calcium absorption: oxalic acid found in spinach, chard, and rhubarb combines with calcium to form insoluble salts which make calcium unavailable; whole grains and beans contain phytic acid, which ties up both calcium and phosphorus. As long as the diet contains varied sources of calcium, however, it is not necessary to be overly concerned about the presence of oxalic acid and phytic acid in these foods.

# RDA

    Infants . . . . . . . . . . . . . . . . . . . . . . . . . . . 360 - 540 mg.
    Children  . . . . . . . . . . . . . . . . . . . . . . . . . . 800 mg.
    Adults . . . . . . . . . . . . . . . . . . . . . . . . . 800 - 1200 mg.

# Functions

- Works with phosphorus to build and maintain bones and teeth and is necessary for normal growth.
- Important for regulating the heart beat and all muscle contractions and nerve transmission.
- Involved in the normal clotting process.
- Maintains permeability of cell membranes.
- Involved in many enzyme systems.
- Necessary for absorption of vitamin $B_{12}$.
- May help prevent premenstrual tension, menstrual cramps, and symptoms associated with menopause.
- May help counteract the harmful effects of radioactive strontium 90.

# Deficiency Symptoms

Prolonged deficiency may result in:
- Osteomalacia and osteoporosis (porous and fragile bones).
- Retarded growth; rickets.
- Tooth decay; bone loss in jaw bones, contributing to periodontal disease.
- Heart palpitations; muscle cramps and spasms; low back pain; joint pain.
- Nervousness, depression, insomnia, and irritability.
- Slow blood clotting; hemorrhaging.

# Toxic Effects

- High levels of calcium in conjunction with a low intake of magnesium and vitamin $B_6$ may cause abnormal deposits of calcium in the soft tissues.
- May prevent coagulation of blood.
- Retarded growth, fatigue.
- Impaired absorption of zinc, iron, and manganese.

# Natural Sources

- Grains — oats, buckwheat, corn tortillas, wheat germ.
- Fruits — oranges, papayas.
- Vegetables — most vegetables, especially dark green leafy vegetables such as collards, mustard greens, endive, lettuce, watercress, kale, cabbage, dandelion greens, beet greens, turnip greens; brussels sprouts, broccoli, okra, green beans, carrots.
- Dairy — milk, cheese, cottage cheese, whey.
- Nuts and seeds — almonds, walnuts, Brazil nuts, hazelnuts, sesame seeds, sunflower seeds.
- Other — tofu, salmon, sardines, kelp, dulse, torula yeast, peanuts, blackstrap molasses, hard water (highly mineralized).

The best food source of calcium is dairy products.

(See Table 3 — BEST FOOD SOURCES OF SELECTED NUTRIENTS, page 142.)

# Chloride

Chloride is an anion which forms compounds with sodium or potassium which are necessary for fluid and electrolyte balance. It is found mostly in gastrointestinal secretions and in the cerebrospinal fluid. Chloride is absorbed in the intestines and excreted in the urine and perspiration. Deficiencies are rare, but may be caused by loss of fluids due to prolonged use of diuretics, or in cases of diarrhea, vomiting, or severe burns. The average dietary intake of chloride is high because of the use of table salt (sodium chloride) and because most foods contain some chloride. Chloride destroys vitamin E and beneficial intestinal bacteria.

## RDA

Estimated Safe and Adequate Intake:
Infants . . . . . . . . . . . . . . . . . . . . . . . . . . . 275 - 1200 mg.
Children . . . . . . . . . . . . . . . . . . . . . . . . . . 500 - 2775 mg.
Adults . . . . . . . . . . . . . . . . . . . . . . . . . . 1700 - 5100 mg.

## Functions

- Necessary for the production of hydrochloric acid, which is involved in protein digestion and mineral assimilation in the stomach.
- Helps the liver remove toxic wastes from the body.
- Helps regulate proper fluid and electrolyte balance in the system.
- Important in the distribution of hormones.

# Deficiency Symptoms

Prolonged deficiency may result in:
- Disturbed fluid and electrolyte balance.
- Impaired digestion.

# Toxic Effects

- Disturbed fluid and electrolyte balance.

# Natural Sources

- Grains — oats, rye, flour.
- Fruits — pineapple, avocados.
- Vegetables — watercress, endive, kale, cabbage, chard, celery, cucumbers, asparagus, tomatoes, beets, radishes.
- Other — table salt, kelp, dulse, seafoods.

The best source of chloride is table salt (sodium chloride).

# Magnesium

Much of the magnesium in the body (60 - 70%) is found in the bones. The remaining 30% is found in the soft tissues and body fluids.

Absorption is regulated by the parathyroid hormone and the amount of calcium and phosphorus in the diet. Phytic acid found in whole grains may prevent absorption of magnesium. Aldosterone, a hormone secreted by the adrenal glands regulates the amount of magnesium excreted in the urine; diuretics and the use of alcohol increase the amount of magnesium lost through the urine. High intakes of fluoride or zinc also increase the urinary excretion of magnesium.

## RDA

Infants . . . . . . . . . . . . . . . . . . . . . . . . . . . . . 50 - 70 mg.
Children . . . . . . . . . . . . . . . . . . . . . . . . . 150 - 250 mg.
Adults . . . . . . . . . . . . . . . . . . . . . . . . . . 350 - 450 mg.

## Functions

- Vital as a catalyst in many enzyme reactions involved in the metabolism of carbohydrates, fats, and proteins.
- Necessary for transmission of nerve impulses and muscle contraction.
- Needed for bone growth.
- Important in the utilization of vitamins B, C, and E.
- Essential for the metabolism of calcium, phosphorus, sodium, and potassium.
- May prevent cardiovascular disease by lowering blood pressure and by preventing a buildup of cholesterol in the arteries.
- Involved in regulating acid-alkaline balance in the body.

- May act as a natural tranquilizer.
- Involved in regulating body temperatures.

## Deficiency Symptoms

Prolonged deficiency may result in:
- Abnormal calcium deposits in the soft tissues.
- Kidney damage and kidney stones.
- Nervous irritability; depression; confusion; disorientation.
- Irregular heart beat; atherosclerosis.
- Muscular tremors; twitching; cramps.

## Toxic Effects

In individuals with kidney disease, excess magnesium may not be excreted adequately, and may produce toxic symptoms such as:
- Diarrhea.
- Unbalanced calcium-magnesium ratio, resulting in depression of the central nervous system.

## Natural Sources

- Grains — wheat, buckwheat, oatmeal, brown rice, millet, rye, wheat bran, wheat germ.
- Fruits — dried fruits, bananas, papayas, berries, cantaloupe, avocados.
- Vegetables — leafy green vegetables, particularly Swiss chard, beet greens, and kelp; alfalfa, green peas, potatoes, yams.
- Dairy — ricotta cheese, whey.
- Nuts and seeds — Brazil nuts, hazelnuts, almonds, cashews, sesame seeds.
- Other — liver, seafoods, legumes, brewer's yeast.

The best food sources of magnesium are whole grains, nuts and seeds, and leafy green vegetables.

(See Table 3 — BEST FOOD SOURCES OF SELECTED NUTRIENTS, page 145.)

# Phosphorus

Phosphorus and calcium, as mineral colleagues, work together and are most effective when present in the proper balance. The bones and teeth contain about 80% of the phosphorus found in the body. The remaining 20% is involved in various chemical reactions within the body.

Phosphorus is more readily absorbed than calcium — 70% of the phosphorus ingested is absorbed, whereas only 30% of dietary calcium is absorbed. Calcium and vitamin D improve the absorption of phosphorus from the intestine; excess iron, magnesium, and antacids interfere with the absorption of phosphorus.

The intake of calcium and phosphorus should be in proper proportion to avoid disturbing the calcium-phosphorus balance. Soft drinks and processed foods and meats are high in phosphorus, but low in calcium, and may interfere with the calcium-phosphorus ratio. Too much phosphorus may lead to increased bone resorption and excretion of calcium.

Some phosphorus in seeds and grains is bound in the form of phytic acid and is unavailable for use by the body. Sprouting the seeds breaks the mineral-phytin bond and releases the minerals for use.

## RDA

Infants . . . . . . . . . . . . . . . . . . . . . . . . . . . . . . . . 240 - 360 mg.
Children . . . . . . . . . . . . . . . . . . . . . . . . . . . . . . . 800 mg.
Adults . . . . . . . . . . . . . . . . . . . . . . . . . . . 800 - 1200 mg.

## Functions

- Involved in the formation of nucleoproteins, phospholipids, vitamin $B_6$, and thiamine.

- Important factor in carbohydrate, fat, and protein metabolism.
- Necessary for growth, repair of tissues, storage and release of energy.
- Involved with calcium, vitamin C, and magnesium in building and maintaining bones and teeth.
- Involved with transmission of nerve impulses and health of the nerves.
- Regulates acid-alkaline balance in the blood.
- Necessary for effectiveness of many of the B vitamins.

# Deficiency Symptoms

Since phosphorus is found in a wide variety of foods, deficiencies are rare. However, in cases of prolonged insufficiency, the following symptoms may appear:

- Loss of appetite; weakness; malaise.
- Poor mineralization of bones and teeth.
- Muscle cramps; joint pain.
- Retarded growth; rickets; periodontal disease.
- Nervous disorders.

# Toxic Effects

A high intake of phosphorus may cause an imbalance in the calcium-phosphorus ratio, creating an adverse affect on the absorption of calcium.

# Natural Sources

- Grains — brown rice, oatmeal, rice bran, wheat bran, wheat germ.
- Fruits — dried fruits.

- Vegetables — corn, winter squash, green leafy vegetables, kale, brussels sprouts, broccoli, green peas, potatoes, sweet potatoes, mushrooms.
- Dairy — milk, cheese, cottage cheese, yogurt, eggs.
- Nuts and seeds — almonds, walnuts, cashews, sunflower seeds, sesame seeds, sprouted seeds.
- Other — liver, brewer's yeast, tofu, fish, legumes, kelp, dulse.

The best sources of phosphorus are liver, brewer's yeast, whole grains, and dairy products.

(See Table 3 — BEST FOOD SOURCES OF SELECTED NUTRIENTS, page 147.)

# Potassium

Potassium, an electrolyte found mostly in the intra-cellular fluid, works with sodium to help control the fluid balance in the cells, and is of primary importance in the maintenance of this balance. It constitutes approximately 0.35% of the body weight.

Aldosterone, the adrenal hormone, regulates the excretion of potassium. However, the use of drugs such as diuretics, cortisone, or aldosterone; extreme diarrhea or vomiting; excessive perspiration; major surgery or injuries; stress; and excessive salt in the diet are among factors that deplete the body of potassium. Potassium is highly soluble and may leach into cooking water, thereby reducing the amount of potassium available from potassium-containing foods.

## RDA

Estimated Safe and Adequate Intake:

Infants . . . . . . . . . . . . . . . . . . . . . . . . . . . 350 - 1275 mg.
Children . . . . . . . . . . . . . . . . . . . . . . . . . . 550 - 3000 mg.
Adults . . . . . . . . . . . . . . . . . . . . . . . . . . . 1875 - 5625 mg.

## Functions

- Maintains fluid and electrolyte balance within the cells.
- Essential for muscle contraction and transmission of nerve impulses.
- Involved in release of energy from carbohydrates, fats, and proteins, and in the formation of glycogen.

- Important in maintaining a normal heart beat.
- Stimulates the kidneys in detoxifying the blood.
- Involved with phosphorus in carrying oxygen to the brain.

# Deficiency Symptoms

Prolonged deficiency may result in:
- Accumulation of sodium in the heart and muscle tissue.
- Impaired glucose metabolism — hypoglycemia.
- Muscular weakness; fatigue; insomnia.
- Irregular heart beat.
- Edema.
- Nervous disorders.
- Weakness of intestinal walls leading to indigestion and constipation.
- Kidney and lung failure.

# Toxic Effects

In kidney disease, the ability of the kidneys to excrete potassium may be impaired, resulting in excess potassium and the following symptoms:
- Abnormal heart rhythm; heart attack.
- Muscle weakness and paralysis.

# Natural Sources

- Grains — buckwheat, millet, rye, wheat bran, rice bran, wheat germ.
- Fruits — all fruits, especially mangos, oranges, bananas, melons, dried fruits, apricots, cherries, papayas, apples, avocados.

- Vegetables — all vegetables, especially green leafy vegetables such as spinach, beet greens, Swiss chard, and broccoli; beets, parsnips, carrots, celery, globe artichokes, mushrooms, winter squash, potatoes (especially the peels).
- Dairy — milk, whey.
- Nuts and seeds — almonds, Brazil nuts, sunflower seeds.
- Other — legumes, mung bean sprouts, dulse, kelp, brewer's yeast, torula yeast, blackstrap molasses.

The best sources of potassium are fruits, vegetables, and whole grains.

(See Table 3 — BEST FOOD SOURCES OF SELECTED NUTRIENTS, page 148.)

# Sodium

Sodium is an essential cation working with potassium and chloride in the extracellular fluid to maintain osmotic equilibrium and fluid volume. The kidneys, regulated by the adrenal hormone aldosterone, are responsible for maintaining the sodium balance of the blood. Excess sodium is excreted in the urine. Deficiencies are rare, because most foods contain some sodium and because of the use of table salt (sodium chloride). The average American diet contains 3-7 grams per day of sodium. However, excessive perspiration, vomiting, diarrhea, or prolonged use of diuretics may deplete the body of sodium and lead to deficiency symptoms.

## RDA

Estimated Safe and Adequate Intake:
Infants ............................... 115 - 750 mg.
Children ............................. 325 - 1800 mg.
Adults .............................. 1100 - 3300 mg.

## Functions

- Works with potassium to maintain proper electrolyte balance and normal fluid levels.
- Maintains a balance between calcium and potassium for normal heart function.
- Necessary for the production of hydrochloric acid in the stomach.
- Regulates the acid-base balance in the body.

# Deficiency Symptoms

Prolonged deficiency may result in:
- Nausea; muscular weakness; cramps.
- Headache; mental apathy.
- Low blood pressure; low blood volume; respiratory failure.

# Toxic Effects

- Edema, dizziness.
- Loss of potassium leading to muscle cramps, fatigue, irregular heart beat.
- Stomach ulcers and cancer.
- High blood pressure; heart disease.

# Natural Sources

- Fruits — cantaloupe.
- Vegetables — celery, celeraic root, carrots, beets, Swiss chard, beet greens, spinach.
- Dairy — milk, cheese, cottage cheese, eggs, whey.
- Other — kelp, seafood, seawater supplements, table salt, blackstrap molasses, brewer's yeast, dulse.

The best sources of sodium are kelp, dairy products, and table salt (sodium chloride).

(See Table 3 — BEST FOOD SOURCES OF SELECTED NUTRIENTS, page 149).

# Sulfur

Sulfur has been called nature's "beauty mineral" because it helps keep the hair, skin, and nails healthy. It is found in all cells as part of the sulfur-containing amino acids methionine, cystine, and cysteine. It is a component of thiamine and biotin, two vitamins in the B-complex. Sulfur occurs widely in nature, but the amount of sulfur present in vegetables and grains depends on the sulfur content of the soil in which they were grown. When the diet contains an adequate amount of protein, the body is probably getting enough sulfur. Vegetarians must be sure to include foods high in sulfur in their diets.

## RDA

None established.

## Functions

- Plays a role in the oxidation-reduction processes.
- Necessary for the synthesis of collagen.
- Used as an ointment, may help treat psoriasis, dermatitis, and eczema.

## Deficiency Symptoms

Prolonged deficiency may result in:
- Brittle nails and hair.
- Dermatitis.

## Toxic Effects

None known.

# Natural Sources

- Vegetables — radishes, turnips, garlic, onions, cabbage, brussels sprouts, kale, horseradish, string beans, watercress.
- Dairy — milk, cheese, eggs.
- Other — wheat germ, legumes, fish, clams.

The best source of sulfur is eggs.

# Part 2

# THE
# MICROMINERALS

# Chromium

Chromium is an essential mineral involved in maintaining a normal glucose metabolism. Marginal deficiencies are common in old age, pregnancy, and protein-calorie malnutrition. Chromium is found in foods in several forms which have varying absorption rates, but overall, less than 3% of the chromium ingested is absorbed. The chromium in brewer's yeast, whole grains, cheese, and liver is more readily available than the chromium in leafy vegetables. Therefore, a varied diet is important to ensure an adequate supply of chromium.

## RDA

Estimated Safe and Adequate Intake:
Infants...........................0.01 - 0.06 mg.
Children..........................0.02 - 0.2 mg.
Adults ...........................0.05 - 0.2 mg.

## Functions

- As an integral part of the glucose tolerance factor, chromium increases the effectiveness of insulin by moving glucose from the blood into the cells.
- Important in the synthesis of cholesterol, fatty acids, and proteins.

## Deficiency Symptoms

Prolonged deficiency may result in:
- Glucose intolerance in diabetes.
- Atherosclerosis.

# Toxic Effects

None known.

# Natural Sources

- Grains — whole grains
- Vegetables — mushrooms, beets.
- Dairy — cheese.
- Other — brewer's yeast, dried beans, peanuts, liver, clams, raw sugar, sugar cane juice, hard water.

The best sources of chromium are whole grains, cheese, and brewer's yeast.

# Cobalt

Cobalt is a mineral essential for the formation of vitamin $B_{12}$. In man, most of the cobalt ingested is not absorbed, and the requirement of cobalt must be taken in as vitamin $B_{12}$. Because it is found mostly in animal sources, vegetarians may not have an adequate supply of cobalt.

## RDA

None established.

## Functions

- Vital part of vitamin $B_{12}$, and necessary for the synthesis of this vitamin.
- Important for the function and maintenance of red blood cells.
- Necessary for the activation of enzyme systems.

## Deficiency Symptoms

Prolonged deficiency may result in:
- Pernicious anemia.
- Slowed growth.
- Nervous disorders.

## Toxic Effects

- Possible enlarged thyroid gland.

# Natural Sources

- Vegetables — minute amounts are found in all green leafy vegetables.
- Dairy — milk.
- Other — seafood, liver, oysters, clams, kelp, seaweed.

The best food sources of cobalt are dairy products, seafood, and liver.

# Copper

Copper is an essential mineral which is widely distributed in food. Very little copper is needed by the body and it is easily obtained in the diet. Deficiencies are rare, but may be caused by protein-calorie malnutrition, sprue, nephrotic syndrome, or prolonged intravenous feeding of a formula low in copper. Copper absorption is increased by the presence of acid and inhibited by calcium. Some copper is stored in the body and could build up to toxic levels. Cooking in unlined copper pots can increase the risk of copper toxicity.

## RDA

Estimated Safe and Adequate Intake:
Infants...............................0.5 - 1.0 mg.
Children............................1.0 - 2.5 mg.
Adults ..............................2.0 - 3.0 mg.

## Functions

- Necessary in order for iron to be absorbed and utilized for the formation of hemoglobin.
- Involved in the production of the nucleic acid, RNA.
- Necessary for protein metabolism and pigmentation of skin and hair.
- Involved with vitamin C in the formation of elastin.
- Present in many enzyme systems.
- Important in the skeletal system, connective tissues, and production of phospholipids.

# Deficiency Symptoms

Prolonged deficiency may result in:

- Anemia due to poor iron absorption.
- Loss of hair; gray hair; skin sores.
- Skeletal defects.

# Toxic Effects

- Nausea and vomiting; diarrhea.
- Headache; weakness.
- Metallic taste.

# Natural Sources

- Grains — buckwheat, rye, barley, oats, brown rice, wheat germ, wheat bran.
- Fruits — dried fruits, mangos, bananas, berries, avocados.
- Vegetables — mushrooms, yams, beets.
- Dairy — milk, eggs.
- Nuts and seeds — Brazil nuts, almonds, pecans, walnuts, hazelnuts, sesame seeds, sunflower seeds.
- Other — oysters, legumes, brewer's yeast, lecithin, seafoods, blackstrap molasses, liver, drinking water.

The best food sources of copper are oysters, nuts and seeds, and legumes.

(See Table 3 — BEST FOOD SOURCES OF SELECTED NUTRIENTS, page 143).

# Fluoride

Fluoride is an essential element found mostly in the bones and tooth enamel, strengthening the bones and making the teeth more resistant to decay. The teeth are affected primarily before eruption, but fluoride may also help prevent periodontal disease and osteoporosis. Fluoride is found in nature as calcium fluoride and is present in all plants, animals, water, and soil. It has been added to drinking water in the form of sodium fluoride for many years in many parts of the world, but there is still controversy over its use since excessive amounts of fluoride are harmful. Fluorosis, characterized by mottling of the teeth, occurs with a fluoride intake of more than 2 - 8 ppm (parts per million).

## RDA

Estimated Safe and Adequate Intake:

Infants. . . . . . . . . . . . . . . . . . . . . . . . . . . . . . 0.1 - 1.0 mg.
Children. . . . . . . . . . . . . . . . . . . . . . . . . . . . . 0.5 - 2.5 mg.
Adults . . . . . . . . . . . . . . . . . . . . . . . . . . . . . . 1.5 - 4.0 mg.

## Functions

- Essential for strong bones and teeth.

## Deficiency Symptoms

- Dental decay.
- Osteoporosis.

# Toxic Effects

- Mottled teeth and brittle bones (fluorosis).
- Calcification of tissues; impaired growth.

# Natural Sources

- Grains — oats, rice, buckwheat, wheat germ.
- Fruits — apples, grapefruit, pears, bananas, cherries.
- Vegetables — carrots, garlic, beet tops, leafy green vegetables, watercress, peas, radishes, corn, eggplant, onions, potatoes.
- Dairy — milk, cheese, butter, eggs.
- Nuts and seeds — almonds, sunflower seeds.
- Other — seafoods, soybeans, fish, seawater, hard water, honey, black tea.

The best source of fluoride is seafoods.

# Iodine

Iodine is essential for the health and function of the thyroid gland. It is converted to iodide in the body and goes to the thyroid gland to become a part of the thyroid hormones thyroxin and triiodothyronine. The remaining iodine ingested is excreted in the urine. The need for iodine is increased during periods of growth, adolescence, pregnancy, lactation, and emotional stress. Certain vegetables — rutabagas, turnips, cabbage, and kale — contain goitrin, which possesses antithyroid activity, thereby interfering with the production of thyroxin.

## RDA

Infants . . . . . . . . . . . . . . . . . . . . . . . . . . . . . 40 - 50 mcg.
Children . . . . . . . . . . . . . . . . . . . . . . . . . 70 - 120 mcg.
Adults . . . . . . . . . . . . . . . . . . . . . . . . . . . . . 150 mcg.

## Functions

- Important in the production of thyroxin and triiodo-thyronine, the thyroid hormones which regulate metabolism, energy production, and the growth rate.
- Involved in the conversion of carotene to vitamin A.
- Helps keep the skin, nails, and hair healthy.

## Deficiency Symptoms

Prolonged deficiency may result in:
- Lethargy; fatigue; low blood pressure.
- Dry skin and hair.

- Obesity.
- Loss of interest in sex.
- Goiter (enlarged thyroid gland) in adults.
- Cretinism in babies born to mothers deficient in iodine — retarded growth, mental retardation, protruding abdomen, swollen features.
- Thyroid cancer.
- High blood cholesterol; heart disease.

# Toxic Effects

- Goiter, from over-worked thyroid gland.
- May impair synthesis of thyroid hormones (hypothyroidism).
- Skin rashes.

# Natural Sources

- Fruits — pineapple, pears, citrus fruits, apples, cranberries.
- Vegetables — Swiss chard, spinach, turnip greens, watercress, garlic, artichokes, potatoes, asparagus, tomatoes, mushrooms.
- Dairy — milk, egg yolks, cheese.
- Fish — Shellfish, haddock, fish liver oils.
- Other — kelp, dulse, other seaweed, iodized salt.

The best source of iodine is seafoods.

# Iron

Iron, the most talked about trace mineral, is also the one most lacking in the American diet. The need for iron increases during rapid growth, pregnancy, lactation, blood loss from surgery, hemorrhage, or heavy menstrual flow, ulcers, and colitis. Newborn infants have sufficient iron stores for six months, after which they must receive iron from their diet. Because iron from animal sources is more readily absorbed than iron from grains and vegetables, strict vegetarians may not be getting enough iron from their diet.

Iron is stored in the liver, spleen, blood, and bone marrow. It is not destroyed or used up, but is recycled. Very little is excreted, and when the need for iron is increased, iron is more efficiently absorbed. Certain substances such as calcium and phosphate salts, phytates, tannic acid in tea, fiber, and antacids decrease the amount of iron absorbed by the body. Vitamin C increases the amount of iron absorbed, and copper is necessary for iron to be utilized.

Older people, who are often lacking in gastric enzymes and hydrochloric acid which are needed for proper assimilation of iron, may become anemic in spite of plentiful iron in the diet.

Iron toxicity can occur with a prolonged excessive oral intake, cirrhosis of the liver, blood transfusions, or an increase in the absorption of iron due to an inborn error of metabolism.

## RDA

Infants . . . . . . . . . . . . . . . . . . . . . . . . . . . . . 10 - 15 mg.
Children . . . . . . . . . . . . . . . . . . . . . . . . . . . . 10 - 15 mg.
Adults . . . . . . . . . . . . . . . . . . . . . . . . . . . . 10 - 18 mg.

## Functions

- Combines with protein and copper for the formation of hemoglobin, the blood component which carries oxygen from the lungs to each cell and removes carbon dioxide.
- Is a constituent of myoglobin, a respiratory pigment in muscle tissue, which also carries oxygen to the cells.
- Necessary in enzymes involved in protein metabolism.

# Deficiency Symptoms

Prolonged deficiency may result in:
- Anemia due to a reduction in the amount of hemoglobin in the red blood cells.
- Pale skin; weakness; fatigue; headache.
- Shortness of breath during exercise.
- Lowered resistance to infection.

# Toxic Effects

- Buildup of iron in the liver, heart, pancreas, and spleen, with resultant damage to these organs.
- Increased susceptibility to infections.
- Grayish skin color.
- Headache; dizziness; shortness of breath; fatigue; weight loss.

# Natural Sources

- Grains — millet, barley, rye, buckwheat, oats, wheat germ, rice bran.
- Fruits — dried fruits such as raisins, figs, apricots, prunes, dates; strawberries.

- Vegetables — turnip greens, spinach, beet greens, Swiss chard, alfalfa, mustard greens, dandelion greens, parsley, beets, Jerusalem artichokes, potatoes, peas, broccoli, carrots, winter squash.
- Dairy — egg yolks.
- Nuts and seeds — black walnuts, almonds, sunflower seeds, sesame seeds.
- Other — liver, tofu, brewer's and torula yeasts, legumes, blackstrap molasses, kelp, dulse, oysters, clams.

The best sources of iron are liver, tofu, brewer's and torula yeasts, whole grains, and green leafy vegetables.

(See Table 3 — BEST FOOD SOURCES OF SELECTED NUTRIENTS, page 144).

# Manganese

Manganese is an essential element in normal bone metabolism and many enzyme reactions. It is widely distributed in plant foods. The amount found in plant sources depends on the amount present in the soil in which they were grown. Much manganese is lost in the processing of foods. Manganese is poorly absorbed from the gastrointestinal tract, and increased intakes of calcium and phosphorus interfere with the absorption of manganese.

## RDA

Estimated Safe and Adequate Intake:

Infants................................0.5 - 1.0 mg.
Children.............................1.0 - 3.0 mg.
Adults ..............................2.5 - 5.0 mg.

## Functions

- Important in several enzyme systems necessary for the metabolism of carbohydrates, fats, and proteins.
- Assists in the transmission of impulses between the brain and nerves and the muscles.
- Involved in the production of sex hormones, thyroxin, and mucopolysaccharides.
- Involved in the activation of vitamin $B_{12}$, synthesis of cholesterol, utilization of choline.
- Necessary for lactation and development of the skeletal system.

# Deficiency Symptoms

Prolonged deficiency may result in:

- Retarded growth; abnormal bone and cartilage development.
- Digestive disturbances.
- Poor reproductive function.
- Impaired glucose tolerance.
- Muscle weakness; lack of coordination; poor equilibrium.

# Toxic Effects

Manganese inhaled as dust or injected may have adverse effects on the central nervous system resulting in weakness, motor difficulties, blurred speech, salivation, and irritability.

# Natural Sources

- Grains — buckwheat, oats, brown rice, barley, bran, wheat germ.
- Fruits — berries, bananas, pineapple, dried peaches, apricots, persimmons, figs, avocados.
- Vegetables — green leafy vegetables such as kale and spinach, green beans, brussels sprouts, beets.
- Nuts and seeds — hazelnuts, Brazil nuts, almonds, walnuts, pecans.
- Dairy — egg yolks.
- Other — liver, oysters.

The best food sources of manganese are whole grains, nuts, and fruits.

(See Table 3 — BEST FOOD SOURCES OF SELECTED NUTRIENTS, page 146).

# Molybdenum

Molybdenum is a trace element that is present in all plants and animals and is essential for plants; it is present in tooth enamel. Molybdenum is easily absorbed, and is a component of several enzyme systems.

## RDA

Estimated Safe and Adequate Intake:

Infants.............................0.03 - 0.08 mg.
Children...........................0.05 - 0.3 mg.
Adults ............................0.15 - 0.5 mg.

## Functions

- Essential part of the enzyme xanthine oxidase, which is necessary for the mobilization of iron from the liver.
- Essential part of the enzyme aldehyde oxidase, which is necessary for the oxidation process.
- Involved in production of uric acid.
- An antagonist to copper, molybdenum may have some protective action in copper poisoning.

## Deficiency Symptoms

None known.

## Toxic Effects

- Diarrhea; anemia; slowed growth.
- Copper deficiency.
- Gout-like symptoms.

## Natural Sources

- Grains — brown rice, millet, buckwheat, wheat germ.
- Vegetables — green beans, dark green vegetables.
- Other — legumes, liver, brewer's yeast, hard water.

The best sources of molybdenum are whole grains and legumes.

# Selenium

Selenium is an essential nutrient with physical and chemical properties similar to sulfur. Deficiencies and toxicity of selenium have been observed in animals, but have not yet been demonstrated in humans. Selenium works closely with vitamin E, and various diseases caused by a combined deficiency of selenium and vitamin E can be treated or prevented by either substance alone. Selenium is a component of glutathione peroxidase, an enzyme which protects the cells from damage by oxidation. The content of selenium in foods depends on the soil in which it was grown, but a varied diet should provide a safe intake of selenium. Heating and processing reduce the amount of selenium in foods.

## RDA

Estimated Safe and Adequate Intake:

Infants...........................0.01 - 0.06 mg.
Children..........................0.02 - 0.2 mg.
Adults ...........................0.05 - 0.2 mg.

## Functions

- A natural antioxidant working closely with vitamin E to preserve tissue elasticity and improve heart function.
- Involved in the production of prostaglandins, providing protection against high blood pressure and heart disease.
- Important in fertility by helping to maintain viable sperm.

- Increases resistance to disease.
- May prevent premature aging by inhibiting the formation of free radicals.
- Helps protect the body against radiation; binds with toxic metals such as mercury and cadmium and prevents them from being absorbed by the body.

# Deficiency Symptoms

Prolonged deficiency may result in:
- Muscle degeneration; heart disease; premature aging.
- May be involved in infertility, crib death, and cancer of the digestive and eliminative tract.

# Toxic Effects

- Gastrointestinal disorders.
- Loss of hair.

# Natural Sources

- Grains — whole grains, wheat germ, wheat bran.
- Vegetables — garlic, mushrooms, broccoli, onions, tomatoes.
- Dairy — milk, eggs.
- Nuts and seeds — Brazil nuts.
- Other — seafoods, liver, brewer's yeast, kelp.

The best sources of selenium are seafoods, liver, and whole grains.

# Silicon

Silicon is present in all connective tissues, and may work with calcium to strengthen bones. The requirement for silicon is easily met by a varied diet.

## RDA

None established.

## Functions

- Present in the skeletal system, tendons, cartilage, and blood vessels.

## Deficiency Symptoms

Prolonged deficiency may result in:
- Poor bone development.
- Osteoporosis.

## Toxic Effects

None known.

## Natural Sources

- Grains — barley, oats, wheat, rye.
- Fruits — apples, strawberries, grapes, raisins.
- Vegetables — beets, onions, parsnips, kelp, cabbage, kale, carrots, potatoes, alfalfa, nettle.
- Dairy — milk.

- Nuts and seeds — almonds, sunflower seeds, flax seeds.
- Other — hard water, peanuts.

The best sources of silicon are hard water and vegetables.

# Zinc

Zinc is an essential trace mineral, with many functions in the human body. Although zinc is readily available in the diet, individuals with liver or kidney disease, gastrointestinal disorders, cystic fibrosis, and extensive burns, as well as alcoholics may be at risk for a zinc deficiency. Stress may increase the need for zinc. The average American diet contains 10-15 grams/day of zinc. Phytates and dietary fiber in vegetables and grains make some zinc unavailable, and in many parts of the United States, the soil has been depleted of zinc. Therefore, vegetarians may need to supplement their diet with zinc. Eating foods that have been stored in galvanized containers may cause a zinc toxicity.

## RDA

Estimated Safe and Adequate Intake:
Infants . . . . . . . . . . . . . . . . . . . . . . . . . . . . . . . 3 - 5 mg.
Children . . . . . . . . . . . . . . . . . . . . . . . . . . . . . 10 mg.
Adults . . . . . . . . . . . . . . . . . . . . . . . . . . . . . . . 15 mg.

## Functions

- Involved in the formation of RNA and DNA and the synthesis of proteins.
- A constituent of many enzyme systems involved in digestion and metabolism.
- Necessary for tissue respiration.
- As a part of insulin is involved in carbohydrate and energy metabolism.

- Necessary for the growth and development of the reproductive system and proper function of the prostate gland; prevention of infertility.
- Speeds up healing of wounds and burns.
- Needed for the absorption of the B-complex vitamins and for the utilization of vitamin A.
- Necessary for the health of the skin, gastro-intestinal tract, and central nervous system.
- Important for normal bone formation and develop-ment of the fetus.
- Involved in the removal of carbon dioxide from the blood through the lungs.

# Deficiency Symptoms

Prolonged deficiency may result in:
- Retarded growth.
- Delayed sexual maturity; enlargement of the prostate gland; infertility; birth defects.
- Increased susceptibility to infections; slow wound healing; skin diseases.
- Stretch marks in the skin; white spots on finger-nails.
- Loss of appetite; poor sense of taste and smell.
- Anemia; lethargy; apathy; fatigue.
- Hair loss, dandruff.
- Atherosclerosis; epilepsy; osteoporosis; poor cir-culation.

# Toxic Effects

- Abdominal pain, nausea, vomiting; bleeding; fever; anemia.
- Premature birth; spontaneous abortions.

- Atherosclerosis.
- Nerve damage.
- Copper deficiency; iron deficiency.
- Increased need for vitamin A.

## Natural Sources

- Grains — oats, brown rice, wheat, cornmeal, popcorn, wheat bran, wheat germ.
- Fruits — most fruits, including mangos, apples, pineapple juice, avocados.
- Vegetables — most vegetables, including green peas, tomatoes, brussels sprouts, mung bean sprouts, green leafy vegetables, spinach, onions, potatoes, mushrooms, asparagus.
- Dairy — milk, cheese, ricotta cheese, eggs.
- Nuts and seeds — Brazil nuts, cashews, hazelnuts, walnuts, pumpkin seeds, sunflower seeds.
- Other — liver, wheat germ oil, brewer's yeast, seafood.

The best sources of zinc are liver, eggs, nuts, and whole grains.

(See Table 3 — BEST FOOD SOURCES OF SELECTED NUTRIENTS, page 150).

# SECTION 3

# VITAMIN & MINERAL
# PURCHASE &
# USE GUIDE

## Natural vs. Synthetic

Vitamins found in nature are never isolated, but are present in the form of vitamin complexes which provide all the nutritive factors in a natural balance. When synthetic vitamins are used, some as yet unidentified or isolated factors may be missing, and the vitamins may be consumed in the wrong proportions.

If natural vitamins are important to you, read the labels carefully. If the label does not specifically say that the vitamin is "natural" or "derived from natural sources," it is most likely synthetic. The words "natural" or "organic" on the label, however, do not necessarily ensure that the vitamins are really made from natural sources. Natural vitamins are usually available only in low potency, and are particularly appropriate for those who do not suffer from any specific disease or deficiency, but are interested in food supplements and vitamins for preventive purposes. The rightful place of synthetic vitamins is in the treatment of acute conditions or severe deficiencies when extremely large doses of easily-soluble and fast-acting vitamins are necessary. The following is a chart to help you in your selection of vitamins:

# Natural and Synthetic Vitamins

| VITAMIN: | IF THE SOURCE GIVEN IS: | IT IS: |
|---|---|---|
| **Fat Soluble** | | |
| Vitamin A | Fish liver oils, lemon grass | Natural |
| | Acetate, palmitate | Synthetic |
| Vitamin D or $D_3$ | fish liver oils | Natural |
| Vitamin D or $D_2$ | Irradiated Ergosterol | Synthetic |
| | Calciferol | Synthetic |
| Vitamin E | Vegetable oil, wheat germ | Natural |
| | Mixed tocopherols | Natural |
| | d-alpha tocopherol | Natural |
| | d-alpha tocopheryl acetate | Co-natural |
| | d-alpha tocopheryl succinate | Co-natural |
| | dl-alpha tocopherol | Synthetic |
| | dl-alpha tocopheryl acetate | Synthetic |
| | dl-alpha tocopheryl succinate | Synthetic |
| Vitamin $K_1$ | alfalfa | Natural |
| $K_2$ | animal source, bacterial culture | Natural |
| $K_3$ | Menadione | Synthetic |
| **Water Soluble** | | |
| Vitamin C | Rose hips, acerola cherries | Natural |
| | Citrus fruits, green peppers | Natural |
| | Calcium ascorbate | Synthetic |
| | Sodium ascorbate | Synthetic |
| | Ascorbic acid | Synthetic |

| | | |
|---|---|---|
| Bioflavonoids | Citrus bioflavonoids, rutin | Natural |
| | hesperidin, citrin | Natural |
| Vitamin B-complex | Brewer's yeast | Natural |
| | Nutritional yeast | Natural |
| | If no source given | Synthetic |
| Vitamin $B_1$ | Yeast or rice bran | Natural |
| (thiamine) | Thiamine Hydrochloride | Synthetic |
| | Thiamine Chloride | Synthetic |
| | Thiamine Mononitrate | Synthetic |
| Vitamin $B_2$ | Yeast or rice bran | Natural |
| (riboflavin) | Riboflavin | Synthetic |
| Vitamin $B_3$ | Yeast or rice bran | Natural |
| (niacin) | Niacin, Niacinamide | Synthetic |
| Vitamin $B_6$ | Yeast or rice bran | Natural |
| (pyridoxine) | Pyridoxine Hydrochloride | Synthetic |
| Vitamin $B_{12}$ | Yeast, liver | Natural |
| | Fermentation concentrate | Natural |
| | Cobalamin, Cyanocobalamin | Natural |
| Biotin | Yeast, liver | Natural |
| | Biotin | Natural |
| | D-biotin | Synthetic |
| Choline | Soybeans, yeast | Natural |
| | Lecithin, liver | Natural |
| | Choline Bitartrate | Synthetic |
| Inositol | Soybeans, corn, yeast, liver | Natural |
| Folic Acid | Yeast, liver | Natural |
| | Pteroylglutamic acid | Synthetic |
| | Folic acid | Synthetic |
| Pantothenic Acid | Yeast, rice bran | Natural |
| | Calcium Pantothenate | Synthetic |
| Para-aminobenzoic | Yeast, liver | Natural |
| acid (PABA) | Para-aminobenzoic acid | Synthetic |

## Some Quick Tips

1. Store vitamins and other supplements in a cool dark place. Exposure to light, heat, and air may reduce the potency.
2. Note the expiration date on the container before purchasing.
3. Use natural supplements when possible.
4. Compare brands and prices for the best buy.
5. Compare the cost per day rather than the cost per tablet or bottle, since potency per tablet may vary.
6. Most food supplements should be taken with meals or immediately after since they are best utilized with foods.
7. Take the fat soluble vitamins (A, D, E, and K) with a meal containing fats.
8. The daily dose of water soluble vitamins should be divided and taken three times a day. The excess beyond immediate needs is excreted in the urine, and therefore must be replaced frequently.
9. Take vitamin E and iron 8 to 12 hours apart. Iron interferes with the utilization of vitamin E.
10. Remember:

    **Water** leaches out vitamin C, B-complex vitamins, and minerals.

    **Heat** destroys vitamin C, thiamine, riboflavin, pyridoxine, folic acid, and vitamin $B_{12}$.

    **Light** destroys vitamins A, C, E, K, $B_{12}$, riboflavin, pyridoxine, and folic acid.

    **Oxidation** destroys vitamins A, C, E, and K, carotene, thiamine, pyridoxine, folic acid, and biotin.

11. Alcohol, aspirin, antibiotics, corticosteroid drugs, mineral oil, and excess sugar in the diet are the most common vitamin antagonists (destroyers).

12. Vitamins and minerals taken during pregnancy and lactation should be according to your doctor's recommendation.
13. If you are suffering from a serious disease or disorder, let your doctor diagnose and evaluate your condition and make recommendations as to vitamin therapy.
14. RDA's are a very general guideline. Let your doctor or nutritionist determine a supplementation program that is best for YOU.

# SECTION 4

# TABLES

Recommended Dietary Allowances

Estimated Safe & Adequate
Daily Dietary Allowances

Best Food Sources

Nutrient Information

Food Compositions

# Table 1

### RECOMMENDED DAILY

*(Designed for the maintenance of good nutrition*

**BASED ON TABLES PUBLISHED BY FOOD AND NUTRITION RESEARCH COUNCIL.**

| | AGE | WEIGHT | | HEIGHT | | PROTEIN | FAT-SOLUBLE VITAMINS | | |
|---|---|---|---|---|---|---|---|---|---|
| | | | | | | | VITAMIN A ACTIVITY | VITAMIN D | VITAMIN E ACTIVITY |
| | From up to years: | kg. | lb. | cm. | in. | Gm | mcg. REª | mcg.ᵇ | mg. ∝ TEᶜ |
| INFANTS | 0.0-0.5 | 6 | 13 | 60 | 24 | kg. x 2.2 | 420 | 10 | 3 |
| | 0.5-1.0 | 9 | 20 | 71 | 28 | kg. x 2.0 | 400 | 10 | 4 |
| CHILDREN | 1-3 | 13 | 29 | 90 | 35 | 23 | 400 | 10 | 5 |
| | 4-6 | 20 | 44 | 112 | 44 | 30 | 500 | 10 | 6 |
| | 7-10 | 28 | 62 | 132 | 52 | 34 | 700 | 10 | 7 |
| MALES | 11-14 | 45 | 99 | 157 | 62 | 45 | 1000 | 10 | 8 |
| | 15-18 | 66 | 145 | 176 | 69 | 56 | 1000 | 10 | 10 |
| | 19-22 | 70 | 154 | 177 | 70 | 56 | 1000 | 7.5 | 10 |
| | 23-50 | 70 | 154 | 178 | 70 | 56 | 1000 | 5 | 10 |
| | 51+ | 70 | 154 | 178 | 70 | 56 | 1000 | 5 | 10 |
| FEMALES | 11-14 | 46 | 101 | 157 | 62 | 46 | 800 | 10 | 8 |
| | 15-18 | 55 | 120 | 163 | 64 | 46 | 800 | 10 | 8 |
| | 19-22 | 55 | 120 | 163 | 64 | 44 | 800 | 7.5 | 8 |
| | 23-50 | 55 | 120 | 163 | 64 | 44 | 800 | 5 | 8 |
| | 51+ | 55 | 120 | 163 | 64 | 44 | 800 | 5 | 8 |
| | Pregnant | | | | | +30 | +200 | +5 | +2 |
| | Lactating | | | | | +20 | +400 | +5 | +3 |

ªRetinol equivalents. 1 retinol equivalent = 1 mcg retinol or 6 mcg beta carotene.

ᵇAs cholecalciferol. 10 mcg. cholecalciferol = 400 IU of vitamin D.

ᶜalpha-tocopherol equivalents. 1 mg. d-alpha tocopherol = 1 alpha ( ∝ ) TE.

ᵈ1 NE (niacin equivalent) is equal to 1 mg. of niacin or 60 mg. of dietary tryptophan.

# DIETARY ALLOWANCES

*of practically all healthy people in the U.S.A.)*

**BOARD, NATIONAL ACADEMY OF SCIENCE, NATIONAL**

Revised 1980.

| WATER-SOLUBLE VITAMINS | | | | | | | MINERALS | | | | | |
|---|---|---|---|---|---|---|---|---|---|---|---|---|
| VITAMIN C | $B_1$ (Thiamine) | $B_2$ (Riboflavin) | $B_3$ (Niacin) | $B_6$ (Pyridoxine) | FOLIC ACID (Felacin) | $B_{12}$ | CALCIUM | PHOSPHORUS | MAGNESIUM | IRON | ZINC | IODINE |
| mg | mg | mg | mg NE | mg | mcg | mcg | mg | mg | mg | mg | mg | mcg |
| 35 | 0.3 | 0.4 | 6 | 0.3 | 30 | 0.5 | 360 | 240 | 50 | 10 | 3 | 40 |
| 35 | 0.5 | 0.6 | 8 | 0.6 | 45 | 1.5 | 540 | 360 | 70 | 15 | 5 | 50 |
| 45 | 0.7 | 0.8 | 9 | 0.9 | 100 | 2.0 | 800 | 800 | 150 | 15 | 10 | 70 |
| 45 | 0.9 | 1.0 | 11 | 1.3 | 200 | 2.5 | 800 | 800 | 200 | 10 | 10 | 90 |
| 45 | 1.2 | 1.4 | 16 | 1.6 | 300 | 3.0 | 800 | 800 | 250 | 10 | 10 | 120 |
| 50 | 1.4 | 1.6 | 18 | 1.8 | 400 | 3.0 | 1,200 | 1,200 | 350 | 18 | 15 | 150 |
| 60 | 1.4 | 1.7 | 18 | 2.0 | 400 | 3.0 | 1,200 | 1,200 | 400 | 18 | 15 | 150 |
| 60 | 1.5 | 1.7 | 19 | 2.2 | 400 | 3.0 | 800 | 800 | 350 | 10 | 15 | 150 |
| 60 | 1.4 | 1.6 | 18 | 2.2 | 400 | 3.0 | 800 | 800 | 350 | 10 | 15 | 150 |
| 60 | 1.2 | 1.4 | 16 | 2.2 | 400 | 3.0 | 800 | 800 | 350 | 10 | 15 | 150 |
| 50 | 1.1 | 1.3 | 15 | 1.8 | 400 | 3.0 | 1,200 | 1,200 | 300 | 18 | 15 | 150 |
| 60 | 1.1 | 1.3 | 14 | 2.0 | 400 | 3.0 | 1,200 | 1,200 | 300 | 18 | 15 | 150 |
| 60 | 1.1 | 1.3 | 14 | 2.0 | 400 | 3.0 | 800 | 800 | 300 | 18 | 15 | 150 |
| 60 | 1.0 | 1.2 | 13 | 2.0 | 400 | 3.0 | 800 | 800 | 300 | 18 | 15 | 150 |
| 60 | 1.0 | 1.2 | 13 | 2.0 | 400 | 3.0 | 800 | 800 | 300 | 10 | 15 | 150 |
| +20 | +0.4 | +0.3 | +2 | +0.6 | +400 | +1.0 | +400 | +400 | +150 | e | +5 | +25 |
| +40 | +0.5 | +0.5 | +5 | +0.5 | +100 | +1.0 | +400 | +400 | +150 | e | +10 | +25 |

eThe increased requirement during pregnancy cannot be met by the iron content of habitual American diets nor by the existing iron stores of many women; therefore the use of 30-60 mg. of supplemental iron is recommended. Iron needs during lactation are not substantially different from those of nonpregnant women, but continued supplementation of the mother for 2-3 months after parturition is advisable in order to replenish stores depleted by pregnancy.

# Table 2

## Estimated Safe and Adequate Daily Dietary Intakes of Selected Vitamins and Minerals[a]

### Vitamins

|  | Age (years) | Vitamin K (mg) | Biotin (mg) | Pantothenic Acid (mg) |
|---|---|---|---|---|
| Infants | 0-0.5 | 12 | 35 | 2 |
|  | 0.5-1 | 10-20 | 50 | 3 |
| Children | 1-3 | 15-30 | 65 | 3 |
| and | 4-6 | 20-40 | 85 | 3-4 |
| Adolescents | 7-10 | 30-60 | 120 | 4-5 |
|  | 11+ | 50-100 | 100-200 | 4-7 |
| Adults |  | 70-140 | 100-200 | 4-7 |

### Trace Elements[b]

|  | Age (years) | Copper (mg) | Manganese (mg) | Fluoride (mg) | Chromium (mg) | Selenium (mg) | Molybdenum (mg) |
|---|---|---|---|---|---|---|---|
| Infants | 0-0.5 | 0.5-0.7 | 0.5-0.7 | 0.1-0.5 | 0.01-0.04 | 0.01-0.04 | 0.03-0.06 |
|  | 0.5-1 | 0.7-1.0 | 0.7-1.0 | 0.2-1.0 | 0.02-0.06 | 0.02-0.06 | 0.04-0.08 |
| Children | 1-3 | 1.0-1.5 | 1.0-1.5 | 0.5-1.5 | 0.02-0.08 | 0.02-0.08 | 0.05-0.1 |
| and | 4-6 | 1.5-2.0 | 1.5-2.0 | 1.0-2.5 | 0.03-0.12 | 0.03-0.12 | 0.06-0.15 |
| Adolescents | 7-10 | 2.0-2.5 | 2.0-3.0 | 1.5-2.5 | 0.05-0.2 | 0.05-0.2 | 0.10-0.3 |
|  | 11+ | 2.0-3.0 | 2.5-5.0 | 1.5-2.5 | 0.05-0.2 | 0.05-0.2 | 0.15-0.5 |
| Adults |  | 2.0-3.0 | 2.5-5.0 | 1.5-4.0 | 0.05-0.2 | 0.05-0.2 | 0.15-0.5 |

### Electrolytes

|  | Age (years) | Sodium (mg) | Potassium (mg) | Chloride (mg) |
|---|---|---|---|---|
| Infants | 0-0.5 | 115-350 | 350-925 | 275-700 |
|  | 0.5-1 | 250-750 | 425-1275 | 400-1200 |
| Children | 1-3 | 325-975 | 550-1650 | 500-1500 |
| and | 4-6 | 450-1350 | 775-2325 | 700-2100 |
| Adolescents | 7-10 | 600-1800 | 1000-3000 | 925-2775 |
|  | 11+ | 900-2700 | 1525-4575 | 1400-4200 |
| Adults |  | 1100-3300 | 1875-5625 | 1700-5100 |

[a]Because there is less information on which to base allowances, these figures are not given in the main table of RDA and are provided here in the form of ranges of recommended intakes.

[b]Since the toxic levels for many trace elements may be only several times usual intakes, the upper levels for the trace elements given in this table should not be habitually exceeded.

# Table 3

## Best Food Sources

# Vitamin A

| Best Food Sources | International Units (I.U.) |
|---|---|
| Beef liver, 3 ounces cooked................................. | 45,390 |
| Calf liver, 3 ounces cooked .............................. | 27,800 |
| Sweet potato, 1 medium boiled in skin .............. | 11,940 |
| Mango, 1 whole ..................................... | 11,090 |
| Cantaloupe, 1/2 ..................................... | 9,240 |
| Carrot, 1 medium raw............................... | 7,930 |
| Pumpkin, 1/2 cup cooked mashed.................. | 7,840 |
| Collard greens, 1/2 cup cooked ..................... | 7,410 |
| Sweet red pepper, 1 medium raw.................... | 7,300 |
| Spinach, 1/2 cup cooked.......................... | 7,290 |
| Dandelion greens, 1/2 cup cooked.................. | 6,145 |
| Turnip greens, 1/2 cup cooked..................... | 4,570 |
| Kale, 1/2 cup cooked .............................. | 4,565 |
| Winter squash, 1/2 cup cooked mashed ............. | 4,305 |
| Mustard greens, 1/2 cup cooked ................... | 4,060 |
| Broccoli, 1 cup cooked............................ | 3,888 |
| Swiss chard, 1/2 cup cooked ...................... | 3,750 |
| Beet greens, 1/2 cup cooked ...................... | 3,700 |
| Apricots, 3 medium raw............................ | 2,890 |
| Papaya, 1 cup cubed .............................. | 2,450 |
| Tomato, 1 medium raw ............................ | 1,350 |
| Asparagus, 1 cup cooked .......................... | 1,220 |
| Egg, 1 large cooked .............................. | 590 |
| Cream cheese, 1 ounce ........................... | 440 |
| Butter, 1 tablespoon............................... | 433 |
| Cheddar cheese, 1 ounce........................... | 370 |
| Milk, 1 cup whole ................................. | 350 |

# Vitamin E

## Best Food Sources

| | Total vitamin E in milligrams (mg.) | Alpha Tocopherol in milligrams (mg.) |
|---|---|---|
| Wheat germ oil, 1 tablespoon . . . . . . . . . . . | 31.82 | 18.68 |
| Soybeans, 1/2 cup dry . . . . . . . . . . . . . . . . | 20.43 | 0.85 |
| Soybean oil, 1 tablespoon . . . . . . . . . . . . . . | 11.72 | 1.37 |
| Sweet potato, 1 medium . . . . . . . . . . . . . . . | 8.17 | 8.10 |
| Almonds, 1/4 cup raw shelled . . . . . . . . . . | 8.16 | 7.98 |
| Sunflower seed oil, 1 Tbsp. . . . . . . . . . . . . . | 7.94 | 7.44 |
| Sesame seeds, 1/4 cup raw . . . . . . . . . . . . . | 7.56 | |
| Corn, 5/8 cup whole, dry . . . . . . . . . . . . . . . | 5.81 | 0.49 |
| Peanuts, 1/4 cup raw shelled. . . . . . . . . . . . | 5.45 | 2.77 |
| Pecans, 1/4 cup raw shelled . . . . . . . . . . . . | 4.96 | 0.31 |
| Whole wheat grain, 5/8 cup. . . . . . . . . . . . . | 4.57 | 1.01 |
| Buckwheat flour, 1/2 cup. . . . . . . . . . . . . . . | 3.95 | 0.16 |
| Rye, whole grain, 5/8 cup . . . . . . . . . . . . . . | 3.80 | 1.28 |
| Rice bran, 1/4 cup. . . . . . . . . . . . . . . . . . . . | 3.73 | |
| Sesame seed oil, 1 Tbsp. . . . . . . . . . . . . . . . | 3.63 | 0.17 |
| Barley, whole grain, 1/2 cup . . . . . . . . . . . . | 2.98 | 0.57 |
| Liver, 3.5 ounces . . . . . . . . . . . . . . . . . . . . . | 2.90 | |
| Sunflower seeds, 1 tablespoon raw, hulled . . . . . . . . . . . . . . . . . . . . . . . | 2.75 | 2.60 |
| Cod liver oil, 1 tablespoon . . . . . . . . . . . . . . | 2.74 | 2.74 |
| Asparagus, 3/4 cup fresh, raw . . . . . . . . . . | 2.10 | 1.98 |
| Oats, 5/8 cup, whole grain. . . . . . . . . . . . . . | 2.05 | 1.09 |
| Brown rice, 1/2 cup raw . . . . . . . . . . . . . . . . | 2.04 | 0.68 |
| Green peas, 1/2 cup fresh, raw . . . . . . . . . . | 1.80 | 0.08 |
| Wheat germ, 1 tablespoon. . . . . . . . . . . . . . | 1.72 | 0.87 |
| Olive oil, 1 tablespoon. . . . . . . . . . . . . . . . . | 1.58 | 1.49 |
| Wheat bran, 1/4 cup. . . . . . . . . . . . . . . . . . . | 1.52 | 0.25 |
| Spinach, 1 cup raw . . . . . . . . . . . . . . . . . . . | 1.50 | 0.94 |
| Apple, 1 medium raw . . . . . . . . . . . . . . . . . . | 0.99 | 0.88 |
| Cabbage, 2/3 cup raw, shredded. . . . . . . . . . . . . . . . . . . . . . . . . | 0.83 | 0.83 |
| Egg, 1 large raw . . . . . . . . . . . . . . . . . . . . . . | 0.53 | 0.35 |
| Butter, 1 tablespoon . . . . . . . . . . . . . . . . . . | 0.22 | 0.22 |
| Milk, 1 cup whole . . . . . . . . . . . . . . . . . . . . . | 0.20 | 0.13 |

# Vitamin B₁ (Thiamine)

## Best Food Sources

| | Milligrams (mg.) |
|---|---|
| Brewer's yeast, 1 ounce | 4.43 |
| Torula yeast, 1 ounce | 3.97 |
| Sunflower seeds, 1/4 cup hulled | 0.71 |
| Rice polishings, 1/4 cup | 0.48 |
| Millet, 1/4 cup raw | 0.42 |
| Soybeans, 1 cup cooked | 0.38 |
| Pinon nuts, 1 ounce shelled | 0.36 |
| Brazil nuts, 1/4 cup shelled | 0.34 |
| Asparagus, 1 cup | 0.24 |
| Beef liver, 3 ounces cooked | 0.22 |
| Green peas, 1/2 cup cooked | 0.22 |
| Rye flour, 1/4 cup | 0.20 |
| Oatmeal, 1 cup cooked | 0.19 |
| Whole wheat flour, 1/4 cup | 0.17 |
| Whole wheat cereal, 1 cup cooked | 0.15 |
| Potato, 1 large baked | 0.15 |
| Buckwheat flour, 1/4 cup | 0.14 |
| Brown rice, 1 cup cooked | 0.13 |
| Lima beans, 1/2 cup dried, cooked | 0.12 |
| Wheat germ, 1 tablespoon | 0.11 |
| Turnip greens, 1/2 cup | 0.11 |
| Wheat bran, 1/4 cup | 0.10 |
| Collard greens, 1/2 cup | 0.10 |
| Milk, 1 cup whole | 0.09 |
| Lentils, 1/2 cup cooked | 0.07 |
| Whole wheat bread, 1 slice | 0.06 |
| Rye bread, 1 slice | 0.05 |
| Whey, 1 tablespoon dry | 0.04 |
| Egg, 1 whole large | 0.04 |
| Sesame seeds, 1 tablespoon | 0.01 |

# Vitamin B₂ (Riboflavin)

## Best Food Sources

| | Milligrams (mg.) |
|---|---|
| Liver, 3 ounces | 13.56 |
| Torula yeast, 1 ounce | 1.43 |
| Brewer's yeast, 1 ounce | 1.21 |
| Cottage cheese, 1 cup creamed large curd | 0.56 |
| Yogurt, 1 cup low fat | 0.44 |
| Milk, 1 cup whole | 0.41 |
| Yams, 1/2 cup | 0.40 |
| Almonds, 1/4 cup raw shelled | 0.32 |
| Broccoli, 1 cup cooked | 0.31 |
| Avocado, 1/2 | 0.23 |
| Millet, 1/4 cup raw | 0.22 |
| Asparagus, 4 large spears cooked | 0.18 |
| Turnip greens, 1/2 cup | 0.17 |
| Whey, 1 tablespoon dry | 0.16 |
| Mushrooms, 1/2 cup raw | 0.16 |
| Soybeans, 1 cup cooked | 0.16 |
| Collard greens, 1/2 cup | 0.14 |
| Egg, 1 large poached | 0.13 |
| Cheddar cheese, 1 ounce | 0.13 |
| Winter squash, 1/2 cup | 0.13 |
| Swiss cheese, 1 ounce | 0.11 |
| Beet greens, 1/2 cup | 0.11 |
| Sunflower seeds, 1/4 cup hulled | 0.08 |
| Wheat germ, 1 tablespoon | 0.05 |
| Wheat bran, 1/4 cup | 0.05 |
| Sesame seeds, 1 tablespoon | 0.01 |

# Vitamin B₃ (Niacin)

| Best Food Sources | Milligrams (mg.) |
|---|---|
| Liver, 3 ounces cooked | 14.0 |
| Torula yeast, 1 ounce | 12.6 |
| Brewer's yeast, 1 ounce | 10.7 |
| Rice polishings, 1/4 cup | 7.4 |
| Wheat bran, 1/4 cup | 3.0 |
| Brown rice, 1 cup cooked | 2.7 |
| Potato, 1 medium baked | 2.7 |
| Mango, 1 | 2.5 |
| Peanut butter, 1 tablespoon | 2.4 |
| Sunflower seeds, 1/4 cup hulled | 1.9 |
| Peaches, 1/2 cup dried, cooked | 1.9 |
| Avocado, 1/2 | 1.8 |
| Green peas, 1/2 cup cooked | 1.8 |
| Cantaloupe, 1/2 | 1.6 |
| Peach, 1 fresh | 1.5 |
| Peanuts, 1 tablespoon | 1.5 |
| Mushrooms, 1/2 cup raw | 1.45 |
| Asparagus, 4 large spears cooked | 1.4 |
| Millet, 1/4 cup raw | 1.31 |
| Apricots, 1/2 cup dried, cooked | 1.25 |
| Almonds, 1/4 cup whole shelled | 1.25 |
| Lentils, 1 cup cooked | 1.2 |
| Broccoli, 1 cup cooked | 1.2 |
| Soybeans, 1 cup cooked | 1.1 |
| Corn, 1/2 cup | 1.05 |
| Kale, 1/2 cup cooked | 0.9 |
| Dates, 5 | 0.9 |
| Collard greens, 1/2 cup | 0.8 |
| Buckwheat flour, 1/2 cup | 0.75 |
| Whole wheat bread, 1 slice | 0.7 |
| Lima beans, 1/2 cup dried, cooked | 0.7 |
| Winter squash, 1/2 cup cooked, mashed | 0.7 |
| Cashews, 1/4 cup | 0.62 |
| Orange, 1 | 0.5 |
| Sesame seeds, 1 tablespoon | 0.4 |
| Wheat germ, 1 tablespoon | 0.3 |
| Milk, 1 cup whole | 0.21 |
| Whey, 1 tablespoon dry | 0.09 |
| Egg, 1 large | 0.03 |

# Vitamin B₆ (Pyridoxine)

## Best Food Sources

| | Milligrams (mg.) |
|---|---|
| Banana, 1 | 0.659 |
| Sunflower seeds, 1/4 cup hulled | 0.45 |
| Sesame seeds, 1/4 cup | 0.315 |
| Cantaloupe, 1/2 | 0.307 |
| Avocado, 1/2 | 0.281 |
| Mango, 1 | 0.277 |
| Wheat germ, 1/4 cup | 0.27 |
| Brussels sprouts, 1 cup | 0.262 |
| Brown rice, 1/4 cup raw | 0.25 |
| Pineapple juice, 1 cup | 0.24 |
| Corn, 1/2 cup | 0.23 |
| Cauliflower, 1 cup | 0.21 |
| Figs, 5 dried | 0.209 |
| Hazelnuts, 1/4 cup | 0.186 |
| Sauerkraut, 1/2 cup | 0.15 |
| Peanuts, 1/4 cup | 0.144 |
| Soy flour, 1/4 cup | 0.12 |
| Wheat bran, 1/4 cup | 0.117 |
| Cabbage, 1 cup | 0.112 |
| Green peas, 1/2 cup | 0.11 |
| Kohlrabi, 1/2 cup | 0.11 |
| Green peppers, 1/2 cup | 0.104 |
| Milk, 1 cup whole | 0.102 |
| Whole wheat flour, 1/4 cup | 0.1 |
| Rye flour (dark), 1/4 cup | 0.091 |
| Cottage cheese, 1/2 cup creamed | 0.07 |
| Egg, 1 large | 0.06 |
| Corn grits, 1 cup cooked | 0.058 |
| Blackstrap molasses, 1 tablespoon | 0.054 |
| Oatmeal, 1 cup cooked | 0.047 |
| Whey, 1 tablespoon dry | 0.044 |
| Whole wheat bread, 1 slice | 0.04 |
| Corn tortilla, 6" diameter | 0.022 |
| Cheddar cheese, 1 ounce | 0.021 |

# Vitamin B$_{12}$

| Best Food Sources | Micrograms (mcg) |
|---|---|
| Liver, 3 ounces | 67.8 |
| Milk, 1 cup whole | 0.871 |
| Yogurt, 1 cup plain | 0.844 |
| Egg, 1 large | 0.773 |
| Cottage cheese, 1/2 cup creamed | 0.59 |
| Swiss cheese, 1 ounce | 0.475 |
| Brie cheese, 1 ounce | 0.408 |
| Brick cheese, 1 ounce | 0.356 |
| Colby cheese, 1 ounce | 0.234 |
| Whey, 1 tablespoon dry | 0.177 |

# Biotin

## Best Food Sources

| | Micrograms (mcg.) |
|---|---|
| Liver, 3 ounces | 81.0 |
| Soy flour, 1/4 cup | 12.0 |
| Peanuts, 1/4 cup | 12.0 |
| Egg, 1 large | 11.0 |
| Walnuts, 1/4 cup | 9.2 |
| Almonds, 1/4 cup | 6.2 |
| Cantaloupe, 1/2 | 6.0 |
| Banana, 1 | 6.0 |
| Mushrooms, 1/2 cup | 5.6 |
| Milk, 1 cup whole | 5.0 |
| Brown rice, 1/4 cup raw | 4.5 |
| Grapefruit, 1/2 | 3.0 |
| Carrots, 1/2 cup | 2.2 |
| Peach, 1 | 2.0 |
| Tomato, 1 medium | 2.0 |
| Blackstrap molasses, 1 tablespoon | 1.8 |
| Apple, 1 | 1.8 |
| Orange, 1 | 1.8 |
| Spinach, 1/2 cup | 1.7 |
| Beet greens, 1/2 cup | 1.5 |
| Elderberries, 1/2 cup | 1.5 |
| Whole wheat flour, 1/4 cup | 1.5 |
| Cauliflower, 1 cup | 1.5 |
| Black currants, 1/2 cup | 1.3 |
| Cheddar cheese, 1 ounce | 1.0 |
| Corn, 1/2 cup | 0.98 |
| Onions, 1/2 cup | 0.76 |
| Buckwheat flour, 1/4 cup | 0.72 |
| Asparagus, 1 cup | 0.67 |
| Cottage cheese, 1/2 cup dry | 0.5 |
| Whole wheat bread, 1 slice | 0.46 |
| Corn flour, 1/4 cup | 0.4 |

# Folic Acid

## Best Food Sources

| | Micrograms (mcg.) |
|---|---|
| Wheat germ, 1/4 cup | 99.5 |
| Avocado, 1/2 | 62.0 |
| Cantaloupe, 1/2 | 45.5 |
| Boysenberries, 1/2 cup | 41.8 |
| Orange, 1 | 39.7 |
| Egg, 1 large | 32.9 |
| Strawberries, 1 cup | 26.4 |
| Banana, 1 | 21.8 |
| Camembert cheese, 1 ounce | 18.0 |
| Brie cheese, 1 ounce | 18.0 |
| Pineapple, 1 cup | 16.4 |
| Cottage cheese, 1/2 cup creamed | 13.0 |
| Milk, 1 cup whole | 12.0 |
| Oatmeal, 1 cup cooked | 9.0 |
| Liver, 3 ounces | 0.186 |
| Beets, 1 cup | 0.126 |
| Asparagus, 1 cup | 0.086 |
| Broccoli, 1 cup | 0.073 |
| Brussels sprouts, 1 cup | 0.056 |
| Spinach, 1/2 cup | 0.053 |
| Green beans, 1 cup | 0.048 |
| Peanuts, 1/4 cup | 0.038 |
| Carrots, 1 cup | 0.037 |
| Pumpkin seeds, 1/4 cup | 0.036 |
| Almonds, 1/4 cup | 0.034 |

# Pantothenic Acid

## Best Food Sources

| | Milligrams (mg.) |
|---|---|
| Liver, 3 ounces | 6.6 |
| Cabbage, 1 cup | 1.14 |
| Cauliflower, 1 cup | 1.0 |
| Avocado, 1/2 | 0.97 |
| Pomegranate, 1 | 0.918 |
| Egg, 1 large | 0.864 |
| Asparagus, 1 cup | 0.837 |
| Mushrooms, 1/2 cup | 0.77 |
| Milk, 1 cup whole | 0.766 |
| Peanuts, 1/4 cup | 0.75 |
| Papaya, 1 | 0.663 |
| Strawberries, 1 cup | 0.507 |
| Brown rice, 1/4 cup raw | 0.5 |
| Sunflower seeds, 1/4 cup hulled | 0.5 |
| Pumpkin, 1/2 cup | 0.5 |
| Oatmeal, 1 cup cooked | 0.468 |
| Cashews, 1/4 cup | 0.45 |
| Green peas, 1/2 cup | 0.45 |
| Pecans, 1/4 cup | 0.42 |
| Rye flour (dark), 1/4 cup | 0.42 |
| Whey, 1 tablespoon dry | 0.419 |
| Wheat bran, 1/4 cup | 0.41 |
| Figs, 5 dried | 0.406 |
| Wheat germ, 1/4 cup | 0.39 |
| Camembert cheese, 1 ounce | 0.387 |
| Hazelnuts, 1/4 cup | 0.38 |
| Corn, 1/2 cup | 0.362 |
| Blackberries, 1 cup | 0.346 |
| Cantaloupe, 1/2 | 0.342 |
| Mango, 1 | 0.331 |
| Whole wheat flour, 1/4 cup | 0.33 |
| Orange, 1 | 0.328 |
| Dates, 5 | 0.323 |
| Soy flour, 1/4 cup | 0.3 |
| Black currants, 1/2 cup | 0.223 |
| Cottage cheese, 1/2 cup | 0.223 |
| Kale, 1/2 cup | 0.19 |
| Whole wheat bread, 1 slice | 0.174 |
| Almonds, 1/4 cup | 0.167 |
| Blackstrap molasses, 1 tablespoon | 0.1 |

# Vitamin C

## Best Food Sources

| | Milligrams (mg.) |
|---|---|
| Guava, 1 medium | 242 |
| Black currants, 1 cup | 200 |
| Red pepper (sweet), 1 medium | 151 |
| Broccoli, 1 cup cooked | 140 |
| Brussels sprouts, 1 cup cooked | 135 |
| Green pepper, 1 medium | 94 |
| Cantaloupe, 1/2 | 90 |
| Strawberries, 1 cup | 88 |
| Mango, 1 | 80 |
| Cauliflower, 1 cup raw | 78 |
| Papaya, 1 cup cubed | 78 |
| Collard greens, 1/2 cup cooked | 73 |
| Kohlrabi, 1 cup cooked | 71 |
| Orange, 1 medium | 66 |
| Persimmon, 1 medium | 66 |
| Kale, 1/2 cup cooked | 51 |
| Turnip greens, 1/2 cup cooked | 50 |
| Asparagus, 1 cup cooked | 45 |
| Grapefruit, 1/2 | 37 |
| Tangerine, 1 large | 31 |
| Potato, 1 large baked | 31 |
| Tomato, 1 medium raw | 28 |
| Cabbage, 1/2 cup raw shredded | 21 |

# Calcium

## Best Food Sources

Milligrams (mg.)

| Food | mg. |
|------|-----|
| Milk, 1 cup whole | 288 |
| Swiss cheese, 1 ounce | 262 |
| Cheddar cheese, 1 ounce | 213 |
| Collard greens, 1/2 cup cooked | 178 |
| Kelp, 1 tablespoon | 156 |
| Blackstrap molasses, 1 tablespoon | 137 |
| Broccoli, 1 cup cooked | 136 |
| Torula yeast, 1 ounce | 120 |
| Cottage cheese, 1/2 cup creamed large curd | 106 |
| Kale, 1/2 cup cooked | 103 |
| Tofu, 3.5 ounces | 100 |
| Mustard greens, 1/2 cup cooked | 96 |
| Almonds, 1/4 cup whole shelled | 83 |
| Dandelion greens, 1/2 cup cooked | 74 |
| Okra, 1/2 cup cooked | 74 |
| Beet greens, 1/2 cup cooked | 72 |
| Hazelnuts, 1/4 cup | 70 |
| Brazil nuts, 1/4 cup raw shelled | 65 |
| Soybeans, 1/2 cup cooked | 65 |
| Corn tortilla, 6" diameter | 60 |
| Whey, 1 tablespoon dry | 59 |
| Orange, 1 medium | 54 |
| Brussels sprouts, 1 cup cooked | 50 |
| Sunflower seeds, 1/4 cup raw, hulled | 44 |
| Sesame seeds, 1/4 cup | 41 |
| Kidney beans, 1/2 cup cooked | 35 |
| Green beans, 1/2 cup cooked | 31 |
| Papaya, 1 cup cubed | 28 |
| Carrots, 1 medium raw | 27 |
| Peanuts, 1/4 cup | 26 |
| Whole wheat bread, 1 slice | 25 |
| Walnuts, 1/4 cup | 25 |
| Buckwheat flour, 1 cup | 23 |

# Copper

## Best Food Sources

| | Milligrams (mg.) |
|---|---|
| Oysters, 3 ounces | 1.30 |
| Oatmeal, 1 cup cooked. | 1.29 |
| Kidney beans, 1 cup cooked | 0.647 |
| Sunflower seeds, 1/4 cup | 0.64 |
| Sesame seeds, 1/4 cup | 0.59 |
| Mushrooms, 1/2 cup | 0.54 |
| Brazil nuts, 1/4 cup. | 0.53 |
| Milk, 1 cup whole | 0.5 |
| Split peas, 1 cup cooked | 0.5 |
| Hazelnuts, 1/4 cup | 0.43 |
| Walnuts, 1/4 cup | 0.35 |
| Figs, 5 dried | 0.292 |
| Almonds, 1/4 cup | 0.29 |
| Blackstrap molasses, 1 tablespoon | 0.284 |
| Pecans, 1/4 cup | 0.28 |
| Avocado, 1/2 | 0.263 |
| Wheat bran, 1/4 cup | 0.25 |
| Mango, 1 | 0.228 |
| Yams, 1/2 cup. | 0.22 |
| Liver, 3 ounces | 0.21 |
| Blackberries, 1 cup | 0.202 |
| Wheat germ, 1/4 cup | 0.175 |
| Buckwheat flour, 1/4 cup | 0.17 |
| Beets, 1/2 cup. | 0.148 |
| Rye flour (dark) 1/4 cup | 0.135 |
| Raisins, 1/4 cup | 0.124 |
| Dates, 5 | 0.119 |
| Banana, 1. | 0.119 |
| Brown rice, 1/4 cup raw. | 0.1 |
| Egg, 1 large | 0.1 |

# Iron

## Best Food Sources

| | Milligrams (mg.) |
|---|---|
| Calf liver, 3 ounces | 12.1 |
| Beef liver, 3 ounces. | 7.5 |
| Torula yeast, 1 ounce | 5.5 |
| Tofu, 3.5 ounces | 5.2 |
| Brewer's yeast, 1 ounce | 4.9 |
| Millet, 1/4 cup raw | 3.9 |
| Pumpkin seeds, 1/2 cup. | 3.9 |
| Blackstrap molasses, 1 tablespoon | 3.2 |
| Lima beans, 1/2 cup dried, cooked. | 2.9 |
| Sunflower seeds, 1/4 cup hulled. | 2.6 |
| Swiss chard, 1/2 cup cooked | 2.6 |
| Soybeans, 1/2 cup cooked | 2.4 |
| Apricots, 1/2 cup dried, cooked | 2.2 |
| Lentils, 1/2 cup cooked | 2.1 |
| Lima beans, 1/2 cup fresh, cooked. | 2.1 |
| Figs, 5 dried | 2.1 |
| Prunes, 5 | 2.0 |
| Spinach, 1/2 cup cooked. | 2.0 |
| Split peas, 1/2 cup cooked | 1.7 |
| Blackeyed peas, 1/2 cup dried, cooked | 1.6 |
| Oatmeal, 1/2 cup cooked. | 1.6 |
| Strawberries, 1 cup whole | 1.5 |
| Beet greens, 1/2 cup cooked. | 1.4 |
| Egg, 1 large poached | 1.2 |
| Dates, 5 | 1.2 |
| Raisins, 1/4 cup | 1.2 |
| Mustard greens, 1/2 cup cooked | 1.2 |
| Buckwheat flour, 1/4 cup | 1.2 |
| Winter squash, 1/2 cup cooked, mashed | 1.1 |
| Rice bran, 1 tablespoon | 1.0 |
| Sesame seeds, 1/4 cup hulled. | 0.9 |
| Corn tortilla, 6" diameter | 0.9 |
| Wheat germ, 1 tablespoon. | 0.5 |

# Magnesium

## Best Food Sources

**Milligrams (mg.)**

| | |
|---|---|
| Kelp, 1 tablespoon | 104 |
| Almonds, 1/4 cup | 96 |
| Cashews, 1/4 cup | 93 |
| Millet, 1/4 cup raw | 92 |
| Wheat germ, 1/4 cup | 90.5 |
| Brazil nuts, 1/4 cup | 87 |
| Hazelnuts, 1/4 cup | 78 |
| Potato, 1 large | 75 |
| Wheat bran, 1/4 cup | 69.7 |
| Sesame seeds, 1/4 cup | 67 |
| Peanuts, 1/4 cup | 63 |
| Oatmeal, 1 cup cooked | 56 |
| Figs, 5 dried | 55 |
| Beet greens, 1/2 cup | 53 |
| Swiss chard, 1/2 cup | 48 |
| Soy flour, 1/4 cup | 44.5 |
| Brown rice, 1/4 cup raw | 43 |
| Turnip greens, 1/2 cup | 43 |
| Collard greens, 1/2 cup | 42 |
| Avocado, 1/2 | 39 |
| Rye flour (dark), 1/4 cup | 37 |
| Whole wheat flour, 1/4 cup | 34 |
| Milk, 1 cup whole | 33 |
| Banana, 1 | 33 |
| Yams, 1/2 cup | 31 |
| Papaya, 1 | 31 |
| Blackberries, 1 cup | 29 |
| Cantaloupe, 1/2 | 28 |
| Green peas, 1/2 cup | 25 |
| Ricotta cheese, part skim, 1/2 cup | 18 |
| Dates, 5 | 14.5 |
| Whey, 1 tablespoon dry | 13 |
| Liver, 3 oz. | 11.1 |

# Manganese

## Best Food Sources

| | Milligrams (mg.) |
|---|---|
| Wheat germ, 1/4 cup | 5.6 |
| Pineapple, 1 cup | 2.55 |
| Blackberries, 1 cup | 1.86 |
| Loganberries, 1 cup | 1.83 |
| Hazelnuts, 1/4 cup | 1.42 |
| Oatmeal, 1 cup cooked | 1.37 |
| Raspberries, 1 cup | 1.24 |
| Brazil nuts, 1/4 cup | 0.97 |
| Brown rice, 1/4 cup | 0.8 |
| Boysenberries, 1 cup | 0.722 |
| Almonds, 1/4 cup | 0.67 |
| Beets, 1/2 cup | 0.63 |
| Persimmon, 1 | 0.596 |
| Peanuts, 1/4 cup | 0.54 |
| Buckwheat flour, 1/4 cup | 0.52 |
| Walnuts, 1/4 cup | 0.45 |
| Strawberries, 1 cup | 0.432 |
| Pecans, 1/4 cup | 0.38 |
| Figs, 5 dried | 0.363 |
| Pears, 5 halves dried | 0.286 |
| Kale, 1/2 cup | 0.25 |
| Avocado, 1/2 | 0.221 |
| Green beans, 1/2 cup | 0.22 |
| Spinach, 1/2 cup | 0.21 |

# Phosphorus

## Best Food Sources

| | Milligrams (mg.) |
|---|---:|
| Brewer's yeast, 1 ounce | 497 |
| Torula yeast, 1 ounce | 486 |
| Calf liver, 3 ounces cooked | 456 |
| Cottage cheese, 1 cup large curd creamed | 342 |
| Sunflower seeds, 1/4 cup raw hulled | 303 |
| Rice bran, 1/4 cup | 290 |
| Milk, 1 cup skim | 247 |
| Yogurt, 1 cup partially skimmed milk | 230 |
| Wheat bran, 1/4 cup | 181 |
| Almonds, 1/4 cup whole shelled | 179 |
| Tofu, 3.5 ounces | 176 |
| Soybeans, 1/2 cup cooked | 161 |
| Swiss cheese, 1 ounce | 160 |
| Lima beans, 1/2 cup dried, cooked | 146 |
| Brown rice, 1 cup cooked | 142 |
| Oatmeal, 1 cup cooked | 137 |
| Cheddar cheese, 1 ounce | 136 |
| Kidney beans, 1/2 cup cooked | 129 |
| Black eyed peas, 1/2 cup cooked | 120 |
| Lentils, 1/2 cup cooked | 119 |
| Brussels sprouts, 1 cup | 112 |
| Walnuts, 1 ounce | 108 |
| Cashews, 1 ounce | 106 |
| Egg, 1 large poached | 103 |
| Lima beans, 1/2 cup fresh, cooked | 103 |
| Potato, 1 medium baked | 101 |
| Broccoli, 1 cup cooked | 96 |
| Dried peas, 1/2 cup cooked | 89 |
| Green peas, 1/2 cup cooked | 79 |
| Corn, 1/2 cup | 73 |
| Whey, 1 tablespoon dry | 70 |
| Wheat germ, 1 tablespoon | 70 |
| Sweet potato, 1 baked in skin | 66 |
| Figs, 5 dried | 64 |
| Whole wheat bread, 1 slice | 57 |
| Winter squash, 1/2 cup cooked, mashed | 49 |
| Sesame seeds, 1 tablespoon raw hulled | 47 |
| Mushrooms, 1/2 cup | 40 |
| Peanuts, 1 tablespoon shelled | 37 |
| Kelp, 1 tablespoon | 34 |
| Kale, 1/2 cup | 32 |

# Potassium

## Best Food Sources

| | Milligrams (mg.) |
|---|---|
| Potato, 1 baked | 782 |
| Kelp, 1 tablespoon | 753 |
| Cantaloupe, 1/2 | 682 |
| Avocado, 1/2 | 680 |
| Blackstrap molasses, 1 tablespoon | 585 |
| Lima beans, 1/2 cup dried, cooked | 581 |
| Torula yeast, 1 ounce | 580 |
| Brewer's yeast, 1 ounce | 537 |
| Soybeans, 1/2 cup cooked | 486 |
| Winter squash, 1/2 cup | 472 |
| Banana, 1 medium | 440 |
| Mango, 1 | 437 |
| Broccoli, 1 cup cooked | 414 |
| Apricots, 1/2 cup dried, cooked | 397 |
| Great northern beans, 1/2 cup cooked | 374 |
| Milk, 1 cup whole | 351 |
| Sunflower seeds, 1/4 cup hulled | 333 |
| Papaya, 1 cup cubed | 328 |
| Apricots, 3 fresh | 301 |
| Globe artichoke, 1 average | 301 |
| Split peas, 1/2 cup cooked | 296 |
| Spinach, 1/2 cup cooked | 291 |
| Almonds, 1/4 cup whole, shelled | 277 |
| Rye flour (dark), 1/4 cup | 275 |
| Orange, 1 medium | 263 |
| Dates, 5 | 254 |
| Peanuts, 1/4 cup | 252 |
| Brazil nuts, 1/4 cup | 250 |
| Millet, 1/4 cup raw | 245 |
| Lentils, 1/2 cup cooked | 244 |
| Beet greens, 1/2 cup cooked | 240 |
| Mung bean sprouts, 1 cup | 234 |
| Swiss chard, 1/2 cup cooked | 232 |
| Prunes, 5 medium | 224 |
| Beets, 2 medium cooked | 208 |
| Peaches, 2 medium raw | 208 |
| Celery, 1/2 cup | 204 |
| Rice bran, 1/4 cup | 187 |

(Potassium, cont.)

## Best food Sources

| | Milligrams (mg.) |
|---|---|
| Carrots, 1/2 cup | 172 |
| Buckwheat flour, 1/4 cup | 164 |
| Wheat bran, 1/4 cup | 159 |
| Whey, 1 tablespoon dry | 155 |
| Apple, 1 medium raw | 152 |
| Mushrooms, 1/2 cup | 146 |
| Fig, 1 large fresh | 126 |
| Wheat germ, 1 tablespoon | 57 |

# Sodium

## Best food Sources

| | Milligrams (mg.) |
|---|---|
| Kelp, 1 tablespoon | 429 |
| Cottage cheese, 1/2 cup creamed | 257 |
| Cheddar cheese, 1 ounce | 198 |
| Egg, 1 large poached | 136 |
| Whole wheat bread, 1 slice | 132 |
| Milk, 1 cup whole | 122 |
| Whey, 1 tablespoon | 80 |
| Swiss chard, 1/2 cup cooked | 63 |
| Beet greens, 1/2 cup cooked | 55 |
| Celery, 1 stalk | 50 |
| Spinach, 1/2 cup cooked | 45 |
| Beets, 2 medium cooked | 43 |
| Carrot, 1 raw | 34 |
| Cantaloupe, 1/2 | 33 |
| Blackstrap molasses, 1 tablespoon | 19 |
| Brewer's yeast, 1 ounce | 10 |

# Zinc

## Best Food Sources

| | Milligrams (mg.) |
|---|---|
| Wheat germ, 1/4 cup | 4.7 |
| Liver, 3 ounces | 3.0 |
| Brazil nuts, 1/4 cup | 1.8 |
| Ricotta cheese, 1/2 cup part skim | 1.6 |
| Cashews, 1/4 cup | 1.5 |
| Lentil sprouts, 1 cup | 1.5 |
| Garbanzos, 1/4 cup dry | 1.4 |
| Wheat bran, 1/4 cup | 1.39 |
| Asparagus, 1 cup | 1.31 |
| Oatmeal, 1 cup cooked | 1.15 |
| Gouda cheese, 1 ounce | 1.11 |
| Buttermilk, 1 cup | 1.03 |
| Hazelnuts, 1/4 cup | 1.0 |
| Lentils, 1/2 cup cooked | 1.0 |
| Sauerkraut, 1/2 cup | 0.94 |
| Milk, 1 cup whole | 0.93 |
| Brown rice, 1/4 cup raw | 0.9 |
| Navy beans, 1/2 cup cooked | 0.9 |
| Mung bean sprouts, 1 cup | 0.9 |
| Cheddar cheese, 1 ounce | 0.88 |
| Whole wheat flour, 1/4 cup | 0.72 |
| Egg, 1 large | 0.72 |
| Green peas, 1/2 cup | 0.6 |
| Raspberries, 1 cup | 0.57 |
| Walnuts, 1/4 cup | 0.56 |
| Brussels sprouts, 1 cup | 0.54 |
| Wheat germ oil, 1 tablespoon | 0.52 |
| Corn meal, 1/4 cup | 0.5 |
| Figs, 5 dried | 0.47 |
| Mushrooms, 1/2 cup | 0.45 |
| Avocado, 1/2 | 0.42 |
| Cantaloupe, 1/2 | 0.41 |
| Onions, 1/2 cup | 0.3 |
| Spinach, 1/2 cup | 0.25 |

# Table 4 NUTRIENT INFORMATION

| Nurtrient | Function | Deficiency Symptoms | Toxicity Symptoms | Food Sources | RDA | Complimentary Nutrients |
|---|---|---|---|---|---|---|
| Vitamin A | Increases resistance to infection. Needed for growth and repair of tissues, night and color vision, healthy skin and eyes. | Night blindness; susceptibility to infections; retarded growth; rough, dry skin; itchy, dry eyes dry dull hair; soft tooth enamel; loss of appetite. | Loss of hair; dry skin; joint and bone pain; loss of appetite; gastrointestinal disturbances; interference with normal growth in children; headaches; fatigue; irritability. | Yellow fruits and vegetables; green leafy vegetables; eggs; butter; liver; fish liver oils. | Infants: 400-420 mcg. RE Children: 400-700 mcg. RE Adults: 800-1000 mcg. RE | Vitamins C, D, E, niacin, pantothenic acid; zinc. |
| Vitamin D | Regulates calcium and phosphorus absorption and metabolism; important for mineralization of bones and teeth. | Rickets—retarded growth in children, with poor bone and tooth formation; osteomalacia; poor assimilation of minerals; reduced parathyroid activity. | Anorexia; nausea; vomiting; excessive thirst and urination; calcification of tissues kidney stones. | Fish liver oils; egg yolks; milk; butter; fish. | Infants and Children: 10 mcg. cholecalciferol (400 I.U.) Adults: 5-10 mcg. cholecalciferol (200-400 I.U.) | Vitamins A, C; fluorine, calcium, phosphorus. |
| Vitamin E | Antioxidant; anticoagulant; maintains circulatory system; protects lungs against pollutants; speeds healing of burns, cuts; prevents scar formation. | Heart disease; reproductive disorders; muscular disorders; fragility of red blood cells | Increased blood pressure; skin rashes; fatigue; weakness. | Wheat germ oil; vegetable oils; wheat germ whole grains; seeds; nuts; some vegetables; legumes; eggs; butter; cheese. | Infants: 3-4 mg. ∝ TE Children: 5-7 mg. ∝ TE Adults: 8-10 mg. ∝ TE | Vitamins A, B₁₂, C; manganese, selenium. |
| Vitamin K | Formation of prothrombin for blood clotting; phosphorylation; bone metabolism; normal liver function. | Hemorrhages; miscarriage. | Synthetic vitamin K may cause jaundice in infants. | Kelp; alfalfa leafy green vegetables fish liver oil; vegetable oil; egg yolks; blackstrap molasses; milk; cheese; liver. | Infants 10-20 mcg. Children: 15-60 mcg. Adults: 70-140 mcg. | Vitamin E. |

151

| Nutrient | Function | Deficiency Symptoms | Toxicity Symptoms | Food Sources | RDA | Complimentary Nutrients |
|---|---|---|---|---|---|---|
| Thiamine (B₁) | Carbohydrate metabolism and energy production; growth and repair of tissues; important for health of nervous system, heart and digestive system; prevents fatigue. | Loss of appetite; impaired hydrochloric acid production; digestive disorders; muscular weakness; irritability; memory loss; fatigue; heart irregularities. | No known toxicity to oral ingestion. | Brewer's yeast; torula yeast; whole grains; seeds; nuts; legumes; milk; eggs; liver; some vegetables. | Infants: 0.3-0.5 mg. Children: 0.7-1.2 mg. Adults: 1.0-1.5 mg. | Vitamins C, E; B-complex; manganese; sulfur. |
| Riboflavin (B₂) | Carbohydrate, fat, and protein metabolism; growth; wound healing; maintains normal red blood cell count; aids cells in utilization of oxygen; protects against pollutants. | Sensitivity to light; eye disorders; cracks and sores in mouth; loss of appetite; digestive disturbances; dermatitis. | None known. | Liver; milk; cheese; eggs; brewer's yeast; torula yeast; wheat germ; whole grains; nuts; green vegetables. | Infants: 0.4-0.6 mg. Children: 0.8-1.4 mg. Adults: 1.2-1.7 mg. | Vitamins A, C, B-complex. |
| Niacin (B₃) | Carbohydrate, fat, and protein metabolism; maintains health of skin, gastrointestinal tract, nervous system; improves circulation. | Poor appetite; digestive disorders; skin lesions; muscular weakness; nervous disorders; dermatitis. | More than 100 mg. may cause release of histamine, causing flushing of the skin. | Brewer's yeast; torula yeast; wheat germ; whole grains; nuts; seeds; liver; fish; eggs; legumes; some vegetables and fruits. | Infants: 6-8 mg. NE Children: 9-16 mg. NE Adults: 13-19 mg. NE | Vitamins C, B-complex; tryptophan. |
| Pyridoxine (B₆) | Carbohydrate, fat, and protein metabolism; necessary for formation of red blood cells and antibodies; regulates balance between sodium and potassium; maintains health of skeletal system, teeth. | Sore mouth, lips, and tongue; dermatitis; anemia; weight loss; weakness; depression; nervousness; kidney stones. | Nervous system dysfunction. | Brewer's yeast; wheat germ; whole grains; nuts; seeds; some fruits and vegetables; milk; eggs; cheese. | Infants: 0.3-0.6 mg. Children: 0.9-1.6 mg. Adults: 1.8-2.2 mg. | Vitamins C, B-complex; magnesium. |

| | Functions | Deficiency Symptoms | Toxicity | Sources | Dosage | Works With |
|---|---|---|---|---|---|---|
| **Vitamin B₁₂** | Carbohydrate, fat, and protein metabolism; nucleic acid metabolism; formation of RNA and DNA; maintains healthy nervous system; necessary for production of red blood cells. | Pernicious anemia; poor appetite; weakness; weight loss; fatigue; retarded growth; loss of memory; depression. | None known. | Liver; milk; fish; eggs; cheese; legumes; seeds; fortified brewer's yeast; wheat germ; oats; spirulina; kelp; whey. | Infants: 0.5-1.5 mcg. Children: 2.0-3.0 mcg. Adults: 3.0 mcg. | Vitamins A, C, B-complex, E; folic acid; iron. |
| **Folic Acid** | Protein metabolism; formation of red blood cells; synthesis of choline; growth. | Anemia; gastrointestinal disorders; inflamed gums and tongue; muscular weakness. | None known. | Green leafy vegetables; legumes; all fruits; Brewer's yeast; whole grains; seeds; nuts; liver; eggs; cheese; milk. | Infants: 30-45 mcg. Children: 100-300 mcg. Adults: 400 mcg. | Vitamins C, B-complex, B₁₂ |
| **Biotin** | Carbohydrate, fat, and protein metabolism; important in metabolism of folic acid and B₁₂. | Loss of appetite; eczema; seborrhea; fatigue; confusion; muscle pain; impaired fat metabolism. | None known. | Brewer's yeast; whole grains; liver; kidney; blackstrap molasses; eggs; milk; cheese; nuts; legumes; most fruits and vegetables. | Infants: 35-50 mcg. Children: 65-120 mcg. Adults: 100-200 mcg. | Vitamins A, C, E₁₂, B-complex, folic acid. |
| **Choline** | Transport of fat soluble substances; health of nervous system; nerve transmission; synthesis of DNA and RNA. | Cirrhosis and fatty infiltration of liver; high blood pressure; atherosclerosis. | None known. | Lecithin; brewer's yeast; wheat germ; liver; fish; egg yolk; legumes; green leafy vegetables; whole grains. | None established. | Vitamins A, B₁₂, B-complex, folic acid, inositol. |
| **Inositol** | Fat and cholesterol metabolism; formation of lecithin; health of heart, liver, kidneys; hair growth. | Constipation; eye abnormalities; high blood cholesterol; eczema and dermatitis. | None known. | Brewer's yeast; wheat germ; lecithin; whole grains; nuts; legumes; citrus; cantaloupe; some vegetables; liver; milk; molasses. | None established. | Vitamins C, E, B-complex, choline. |

| Nutrient | Function | Deficiency Symptoms | Toxicity Symptoms | Food Sources | RDA | Complimentary Nutrients |
|---|---|---|---|---|---|---|
| **Pantothenic Acid** | Release of energy from carbohydrates, proteins, and fats; improves production of cortisone and other adrenal hormones; anti-stress factor; increases resistance to infection; synthesis of fats. | Fatigue; decreased resistance to infection; gastrointestinal disturbances; depression; irritability. | None known. | Brewer's yeast; whole grains; liver; eggs; milk; legumes; nuts; seeds; vegetables; fruits. | Infants: 2-3 mg. Children: 3-5 mg. Adults: 4-7 mg. | Vitamins C, B-complex, biotin, folic acid. |
| **Para-aminobenzoic Acid** | Involved in production of folic acid and formation of red blood cells; protects skin from sunburn. | Fatigue; irritability; depression; anemia; eczema; gray hair; reproductive disorders. | Nausea and vomiting. | Brewer's yeast; whole grains; milk; eggs; liver; sunflower seeds; molasses; mushrooms. | None established. | Vitamins C, B-complex, folic acid. |
| **Vitamin C** | Synthesis and health of collagen; strengthens all connective tissues — skin, bones, teeth, joints, muscles and tendons, cartilage, capillaries; increased resistance to infection; improves absorption of iron; promotes healing of wounds; helps cope with stress. | Tooth decay; periodontal disease; slow healing of wounds; lowered resistance to infections; weakness; fatigue; bleeding gums; hemorrhage in joints and skin; aching bones, joints, muscles. | Skin rashes; diarrhea; excessive urination; false positive tests for glucosuria. | Red and green peppers; cabbage; broccoli; brussels sprouts; potatoes; tomatoes; papaya; guavas; citrus; mangos; persimmon; berries; black currants. | Infants: 35 mg. Children: 45 mg. Adults: 60 mg. | Bioflavonoids, Vitamins A, B₆, pantothenic acid; calcium, magnesium. |
| **Bioflavonoids** | Strengthen capillary walls; enhance absorption and utilization of vitamin C. | Capillary fragility; susceptibility to hemorrhages and bruises. | None known. | Citrus; grapes; apricots; berries; black currants; prunes; rose hips; green peppers; buckwheat. | None established. | Vitamin C. |

154

| Mineral | Functions | Deficiency Symptoms | Excess Symptoms | Food Sources | Amounts | Works With |
|---|---|---|---|---|---|---|
| **Calcium** | Builds and maintains bones and teeth; regulates heart beat, muscle contractions, and nerve transmissions; involved in normal blood clotting. | Porous and fragile bones; tooth decay; bone loss in jaws; retarded growth; rickets; muscle and joint pain; slow blood clotting; nervousness; depression; insomnia; irritability. | Abnormal deposits of calcium in soft tissues; retarded growth; fatigue; impaired absorption of zinc, iron, and manganese. | Milk; cheese; whey; tofu; salmon; sardines; dark green leafy vegetables; legumes; seeds; nuts; whole grains; hard water; blackstrap molasses. | Infants: 360-540 mg. Children: 800 mg. Adults: 800-1200 mg. | Vitamins A, C, D; phosphorus, magnesium. |
| **Phosphorus** | Building and maintenance of bones and teeth; involved in formation of nucleoproteins, phospholipids, vitamin $B_6$, and thiamine; important in carbohydrate, fat, and protein metabolism, transmission of nerve impulses. | Loss of appetite; weakness; poor mineralization of bones and teeth; muscle cramps; joint pain; retarded growth; rickets; periodontal disease; nervous disorders. | Imbalance in calcium-phosphorus ratio. | Milk; cheese; tofu; fish; seeds; nuts; whole grains; dried fruits; green leafy vegetables; winter squash; potatoes. | Infants: 210-360 mg. Children: 800 mg. Adults: 800-1200 mg. | Vitamins A, D; calcium. |
| **Magnesium** | Catalyst in enzyme reactions involving metabolism of carbohydrates, fats, and proteins; involved in transmission of nerve impulses and muscle contractions, bone growth, metabolism of calcium, phosphorus, sodium, and potassium. | Abnormal calcium deposits in soft tissues; kidney damage; kidney stones; nervousness; depression; confusion; muscle tremors. | Diarrhea; unbalanced calcium-magnesium ratio. | Kelp; wheat germ; whole grains; legumes; seeds; nuts; green leafy vegetables; seafoods; dried fruits; whey; liver. | Infants: 50-70 mg. Children: 150-250 mg. Adults: 300-400 mg. | Vitamins C, $B_6$; calcium, phosphorus. |

| Nurtrient | Function | Deficiency Symptoms | Toxicity Symptoms | Food Sources | RDA | Complimentary Nutrients |
|---|---|---|---|---|---|---|
| Potassium | Maintains fluid and electrolyte balance in cells; involved in muscle contraction and transmission of nerve impulses; involved in release of energy from protein, carbohydrates, and fats; maintains normal heartbeat. | Accumulation of sodium in heart and muscle tissue; impaired glucose metabolism; muscle weakness; fatigue; insomnia; irregular heartbeat; nervous disorders; constipation. | Abnormal heart rhythm; heart attack; muscle weakness; paralysis. | All vegetables, especially green leafy vegetables; legumes; all fruits, especially mangos, oranges, bananas, melons, dried fruits; whole grains; brewer's yeast; blackstrap molasses; milk; whey; seeds; nuts. | Infants: 350-1275 mg. Children: 550-3000 mg. Adults: 1875-5625 mg. | Vitamin B₆; magnesium. |
| Sulfur | Part of the amino acids methionine, cystine, and cysteine; keeps hair, skin, nails healthy; involved in oxidation reduction process; necessary for synthesis of collagen; component of thiamine and biotin. | Brittle hair and nails; skin disorders. | None known. | Radishes; turnips; garlic; onions; cabbage; brussels sprouts; kale; horseradish; string beans; watercress; legumes; wheat germ; fish; eggs; clams. | None established. | B-complex. |
| Chloride | Necessary for production of hydrochloric acid; helps regulate fluid and electrolyte balance; important in distribution of hormones; helps liver remove toxic wastes. | Disturbed fluid and electrolyte balance; impaired digestion. | Disturbed fluid and electrolyte balance. | Kelp; dulse; watercress; endive; kale; cabbage; chard; celery; avocados; tomatoes; beets; radishes; asparagus; pineapple; oats; rye; seafood; sea salt. | Infants: 275-1200 mg. Children: 500-2775 mg. Adults: 1700-5100 mg. | |

| | Function | Deficiency Symptoms | Toxicity/Excess | Sources | Amounts | Works With |
|---|---|---|---|---|---|---|
| **Sodium** | Maintains electrolyte balance and normal fluid levels; necessary for production of hydrochloric acid. | Nausea; muscle weakness; cramps; headache; low blood pressure. | Edema; dizziness; loss of potassium leading to muscle cramps, fatigue, irregular heartbeat; stomach ulcers and cancer; high blood pressure; heart disease. | Celery; celeriac root; carrots; beets; Swiss chard; beet greens; spinach; seafood; milk; cheese whey; cottage cheese; sea salt; cantaloupe; blackstrap molasses; brewer's yeast; kelp; dulse. | Infants: 115-750 mg. Children: 325-1800 mg. Adults: 1100-3300 mg. | |
| **Iron** | Necessary for formation of hemoglobin and myoglobin; involved in protein metabolism. | Anemia; pale skin; weakness; fatigue; shortness of breath; lowered resistance to infections. | Build up of iron in liver and spleen with resultant damage to these organs; increased susceptibility to infection. | Liver; egg yolks; tofu; blackstrap molasses; brewer's yeast; torula yeast; kelp; whole grains; dried fruits; green leafy vegetables; legumes; nuts; seeds. | Infants: 10-15 mg. Children: 10-15 mg. Adults: 10-18 mg. | Vitamins C, B6, B12, folic acid. |
| **Zinc** | Involved in formation of RNA and DNA and synthesis of proteins; constituent of many enzyme systems, insulin; speeds up healing of wounds; important in health of skin, gastrointestinal tract, central nervous system, bone formation, development of fetus, development of reproductive system, and prostate gland function. | Retarded growth; delayed sexual maturity; increased susceptibility to infections; stretch marks on skin; loss of appetite; poor sense of smell and taste; anemia; fatigue. | Abdominal pain; nausea; vomiting; premature birth; atherosclerosis; nerve damage; copper and iron deficiency; increased need for vitamin A | Whole grains; most vegetables and fruits; nuts; seeds; milk; cheese; egg yolks; liver. | Infants: 3-5 mg. Children: 10 mg. Adults: 15 mg. | Vitamins A, C, D. |

| Nurtrient | Function | Deficiency Symptoms | Toxicity Symptoms | Food Sources | RDA | Complimentary Nutrients |
|---|---|---|---|---|---|---|
| Iodine | Important in production of thyroxine and prevention of goiter; regulation of metabolism, energy production, and growth rate; involved in conversion of carotene to vitamin A. | Enlarged thyroid gland (goiter); lethargy; fatigue; dry skin and hair; cretenism in babies born to mothers deficient in iodine. | Goiter; hypothyroidism; skin rashes. | Kelp; Swiss chard; spinach; turnip greens; watercress; garlic; citrus fruits; pineapple; egg yolks; shellfish; fish liver oils; iodized salt. | Infants: 40-50 mcg. Children: 70-120 mcg. Adults: 150 mcg. | |
| Copper | Needed for absorption and utilization of iron; involved in production of DNA, protein metabolism; present in many enzyme systems. | Anemia due to poor iron absorption; skeletal defects; loss of hair; skin sores. | Nausea; vomiting; diarrhea; headache; weakness; metalic taste. | Nuts; seeds; legumes; whole grains; lecithin; blackstrap molasses; mushrooms; yams; beets; avocados; dried fruits; mangos; bananas; sea foods; eggs; milk. | Infants: 0.5-1.0 mg. Children: 1.0-2.5 mg. Adults: 2.0-3.0 mg. | Iron, cobalt. |
| Manganese | Necessary for metabolism of carbohydrates, fats, proteins; involved in transmissions of nerve impulses, production of hormones; development of skeletal system. | Retarded growth; abnormal skeletal development; digestive disturbances; poor reproductive function; impaired glucose tolerance; muscle weakness. | Weakness; motor difficulties; blurred speech; salivation; irritability. | Green leafy vegetables; fruits; nuts; whole grains; liver; egg yolks. | Infants: 0.5-1.0 mg. Children: 1.0-3.0 mg. Adults: 2.5-5.0 mg. | Vitamins E, thiamine; calcium; phosphorus. |
| Fluoride | Essential for strong bones and teeth. | Dental decay; osteoporosis | Fluorosis — mottled teeth and brittle bones; calcification of tissues; impaired growth. | Whole grains; legumes; nuts; seeds; milk; cheese; fish; eggs; vegetables; hard water; black tea; fruits. | Infants: 0.1-1.0 mg. Children: 0.5-2.5 mg. Adults: 1.5-4.0 mg. | |

158

| Mineral | Function | Deficiency | Toxicity | Sources | Recommended amounts | Interacts with |
|---|---|---|---|---|---|---|
| **Chromium** | Increases effectiveness of insulin; important in synthesis of cholesterol, fatty acids and proteins. | Glucose intolerance in diabetics; atherosclerosis. | None known. | Whole grains; brewer's yeast; legumes; mushrooms; liver; cheese; clams; hard water. | Infants: 0.01–0.06 mg. Children: 0.02–0.2 mg. Adults: 0.05–0.2 mg. | |
| **Selenium** | An antioxidant working closely with vitamin E. Involved in production of prostaglandins, proper heart function; a component of glutathione peroxidase; binds with toxic metals. | Muscle degeneration; heart disease; premature aging; infertility; crib death. | Gastrointestinal disorders; loss of hair. | Brewer's yeast; kelp; wheat germ; whole grains; garlic; mushrooms; broccoli; onions; tomatoes; milk; eggs; liver; Brazil nuts. | Infants: 0.01–0.06 mg. Children: 0.02–0.2 mg. Adults: 0.05–0.2 mg. | Vitamin E. |
| **Molybdenum** | Involved in oxidation process, production of uric acid. | None demonstrated in humans. | Diarrhea; anemia; slowed growth; copper deficiency; gout-like symptoms. | Brewer's yeast; wheat germ; whole grains; legumes; dark green vegetables; liver; hard water. | Infants: 0.03–0.08 mg. Children: 0.06–0.3 mg. Adults: 0.15–0.5 mg. | |
| **Silicon** | Present in skeletal system, tendons, cartilage, and blood vessels. | Poor bone development and osteoporosis. | None known. | Green leafy vegetables; seeds; nuts; peanuts; whole grains; milk; hard water; fruits. | None established. | |
| **Cobalt** | Vital part of vitamin B₁₂; involved in maintenance of red blood cells, activation of enzyme systems | Pernicious anemia; slow growth; nervous disorders. | Possible enlarged thyroid. | Liver; oysters; clams; milk; green leafy vegetables; kelp; sea weed. | None established. | Copper, iron, zinc. |

# Table 5

## COMPOSITION OF FOODS
### 100 grams, edible portion

(dash (—) denotes lack of reliable data for a constituent believed to be present in measurable amount)

| FOOD | CALORIES | PROTEINS grams | FATS grams | CARBOHYDRATES grams | CALCIUM mg. | PHOSPHORUS mg. | MAGNESIUM mg. | IRON mg. | SODIUM mg. | POTASSIUM mg. | VITAMIN A VALUE IU | B₁ mg. | B₂ mg. | NIACIN mg. | VITAMIN C mg. |
|---|---|---|---|---|---|---|---|---|---|---|---|---|---|---|---|
| ACEROLA cherry, raw | 28 | .4 | .3 | 6.8 | 12 | 11 | — | .2 | 8 | 83 | — | .02 | .06 | 0.4 | 1,300 |
| ACEROLA JUICE, raw | 23 | .4 | .3 | 4.8 | 10 | 9 | — | .5 | 3 | — | — | .02 | .06 | .4 | 1,600 |
| ALMONDS, dried | 598 | 18.6 | 54.2 | 19.5 | 234 | 504 | 270 | 4.7 | 4 | 773 | 0 | .24 | .92 | 3.5 | trace |
| APPLES, freshly harvested | 58 | .2 | .6 | 14.5 | 7 | 10 | 8 | .3 | 1 | 110 | 90 | .03 | .02 | .4 | 7-20 |
| APPLE JUICE, canned or bottled | 47 | .1 | trace | 11.9 | 6 | 9 | 4 | .6 | 1 | 101 | — | .01 | .02 | .1 | 1 |
| APRICOTS, raw | 51 | 1.0 | .2 | 12.8 | 17 | 23 | 12 | .5 | 1 | 281 | 2,700 | .03 | .04 | .6 | 10 |
| APRICOTS, dried, uncooked | 260 | 5.0 | .5 | 66.5 | 67 | 108 | 62 | 5.5 | 26 | 979 | 10,900 | .01 | .16 | 3.3 | 12 |
| ARTICHOKES, globe or French, raw | 9-47 | 2.9 | 0.2 | 10.6 | 51 | 88 | — | 1.3 | 43 | 430 | 160 | .08 | .05 | 1.0 | 12 |
| cooked | 8-44 | 2.8 | .2 | 9.6 | 51 | 68 | — | 1.1 | 30 | 301 | 150 | .07 | .04 | .7 | 8 |
| ARTICHOKES, Jerusalem, raw | 7-75 | 2.3 | .1 | 16.7 | 14 | 78 | 11 | 3.4 | — | — | 20 | .2 | .06 | 1.3 | 4 |
| ASPARAGUS, raw spears | 26 | 2.5 | .2 | 5.0 | 22 | 62 | 20 | 1.0 | 2 | 278 | 900 | .18 | .20 | 1.5 | 33 |
| cooked spears | 20 | 2.2 | .2 | 3.6 | 21 | 50 | 14 | .6 | 1 | 183 | 900 | .16 | .18 | 1.4 | 26 |
| AVOCADOS, raw | 167 | 2.1 | 16.4 | 6.3 | 10 | 42 | 45 | .6 | 4 | 604 | 290 | .11 | .20 | 1.6 | 14 |
| BANANAS, common, raw | 85 | 1.1 | .2 | 22.2 | 8 | 26 | 33 | .7 | 1 | 370 | 190 | .05 | .06 | .7 | 10 |
| BARLEY, pearled, light | 349 | 8.2 | 1.0 | 78.8 | 16 | 189 | 37 | 2.0 | 3 | 160 | 0 | .12 | .05 | 3.1 | 0 |

|  | | | | | | | | | | | | | | | |
|---|---|---|---|---|---|---|---|---|---|---|---|---|---|---|---|
| BEANS, common white, cooked | 118 | 7.8 | .6 | 21.2 | 50 | 148 | 37 | 2.7 | 7 | 416 | 0 | .14 | .07 | .7 | 0 |
| red, cooked | 347 | 7.8 | .5 | 21.4 | 38 | 140 |  | 2.7 | 3 | 340 | trace | .11 | .06 | .7 |  |
| pinto, raw | 349 | 22.9 | 1.2 | 63.7 | 135 | 457 |  | 6.4 | 10 | 984 |  | .84 | .21 | 2.2 |  |
| lima, immature cooked | 123 | 8.4 | .5 | 22.1 | 52 | 142 | 46 | 2.8 | 2 | 650 | 290 | .24 | .12 | 1.4 | 29 |
| lima, mature, cooked | 138 | 8.2 | .6 | 25.6 | 29 | 154 | 48 | 3.1 | 2 | 612 | 20 | .13 | .06 | .7 | 19 |
| mung, sprouted, raw | 38 | 3.8 | .2 | 6.6 | 19 | 64 |  | 1.3 | 5 | 223 |  | .13 | .13 | .8 | 19 |
| green, raw | 32 | 1.9 | .2 | 7.1 | 56 | 44 | 32 | .6 | 7 | 243 | 600 | .8 | .11 | .5 | 12 |
| green, cooked | 25 | 1.6 | .2 | 5.4 | 50 | 37 | 21 | .7 | 4 | 151 | 540 | .07 | .09 | .5 | 10 |
| BEETS, red, raw | 43 | 1.5 | .1 | 9.9 | 16 | 33 | 25 | .5 | 60 | 335 | 20 | .03 | .05 | .4 | 6 |
| red, cooked | 32 | 1.1 | .1 | 7.2 | 14 | 23 | 15 |  | 43 | 208 | 20 | .03 | .04 | .3 |  |
| BEET GREENS, raw | 24 | 2.2 | .3 | 4.6 | 119 | 40 | 106 | 3.3 | 130 | 570 | 6,100 | .10 | .22 | .4 | 30 |
| cooked | 18 | 1.7 | .2 | 3.3 | 99 | 25 |  | 1.9 | 76 | 332 | 5,000 | .07 | .15 | .3 | 15 |
| BLACKBERRIES, raw | 58 | 1.2 | .9 | 12.9 | 32 | 19 | 30 | .9 | 1 | 170 | 200 | .03 | .04 | .4 | 21 |
| BLUEBERRIES, raw | 62 | .7 | .5 | 15.3 | 15 | 13 | 6 | 1.0 | 1 | 81 | 100 | .03 | .06 | .5 | 14 |
| BRAZIL NUTS, raw | 654 | 14.3 | 66.9 | 10.9 | 186 | 693 | 225 | 3.4 | 1 | 715 | trace | .96 | .12 | 1.6 |  |
| BROCCOLI, raw spears | 32 | 3.6 | .3 | 5.9 | 103 | 78 | 24 | 1.1 | 15 | 382 | 2,500 | .10 | .23 | .9 | 113 |
| cooked | 26 | 3.1 | .3 | 4.5 | 88 | 62 | 21 | .8 | 10 | 267 | 2,500 | .09 | .20 | .8 | 90 |
| BRUSSELS SPROUTS, raw | 45 | 4.9 | .4 | 8.3 | 36 | 80 | 29 | 1.5 | 14 | 390 | 550 | .10 | .16 | .9 | 102 |
| cooked | 36 | 4.2 | .4 | 6.4 | 32 | 72 | 21 | 1.1 | 10 | 273 | 520 | .08 | .14 | .8 | 87 |
| BUCKWHEAT, whole grain | 335 | 11.7 | 2.4 | 72.9 | 114 | 282 | 229 | 3.1 |  | 448 | 0 | .60 | .18 | 4.4 | 0 |
| BUTTER, salted | 716 | .6 | 81. | .4 | 20 | 16 |  | 0 | 987 | 23 | 3,300 |  |  |  | 0 |
| unsalted | 720 | .6 | 82. | .4 | 20 | 16 |  | 0 | 8 | 9 | 3,350 |  |  |  |  |
| BUTTERMILK, cultured, from skim milk | 36 | 3.6 | .1 | 5.1 | 121 | 95 | 14 | trace | 130 | 140 | trace | 0.4 | .05 | .1 | 1 |
| CABBAGE, white, raw | 24 | 1.3 | .2 | 5.4 | 49 | 29 | 13 | .4 | 20 | 233 | 130 | .05 | .06 | .3 | 47 |
| red, raw | 31 | 2.0 | .2 | 6.9 | 42 | 35 |  | .8 | 26 | 268 | 40 | .09 | .08 | .4 | 61 |
| savoy, raw | 24 | 2.4 | .2 | 4.6 | 67 | 54 |  | .9 | 22 | 269 | 200 | .05 | .05 | .3 | 55 |
| CAROB FLOUR | 180 | 4.5 | 1.4 | 80.7 | 352 | 81 |  |  |  |  |  |  |  |  |  |
| CARROTS, raw | 42 | 1.1 | .2 | 9.7 | 37 | 36 | 23 | .7 | 47 | 341 | 11,000 | .06 |  | .6 | 8 |
| CASHEW NUTS | 561 | 17.2 | 45.7 | 29.3 | 38 | 373 | 267 | 3.8 | 15 | 464 | 100 | .43 | .25 | 1.8 |  |
| CALIFLOWER, raw | 27 | 2.7 | .2 | 5.2 | 25 | 56 | 24 | 1.1 | 13 | 295 | 60 | .11 | .10 | .7 | 78 |
| cooked | 22 | 2.3 | .2 | 4.1 | 21 | 42 |  | .7 | 9 | 206 | 60 | .09 | .08 | .6 | 55 |
| CELERY, raw | 17 | .9 | .1 | 3.9 | 39 | 28 | 22 | .3 | 126 | 341 | 240 | .03 | .03 | .8 | 9 |
| CHARD, Swiss, raw | 25 | 2.4 | 0.3 | 4.6 | 88 | 39 | 65 | 3.2 | 147 | 550 | 6,500 | .06 | .17 | .5 | 32 |
| cooked | 18 | 1.8 | .2 | 3.3 | 73 | 24 |  | 1.8 | 86 | 321 | 5,400 | .04 | .11 | .4 | 16 |

| FOOD | CALORIES | PROTEINS grams | FATS grams | CARBOHYDRATES grams | CALCIUM mg. | PHOSPHORUS mg. | MAGNESIUM mg. | IRON mg. | SODIUM mg. | POTASSIUM mg. | VITAMIN A VALUE IU | B1 mg. | B2 mg. | NIACIN mg. | VITAMIN C mg. |
|---|---|---|---|---|---|---|---|---|---|---|---|---|---|---|---|
| CHEESE, Blue or Roquefort | 368 | 21.5 | 30.5 | 2.0 | 315 | 339 | 48 | .5 | 700 | 82 | 1,240 | .03 | .61 | 1.2 | |
| Cheddar | 398 | 25.0 | 32.2 | 2.1 | 750 | 478 | 45 | 1.0 | 229 | 85 | 1,310 | .03 | .46 | .1 | |
| Cottage, creamed | 106 | 13.6 | 4.2 | 2.9 | 94 | 152 | | .3 | 290 | 72 | 170 | .03 | .25 | .1 | |
| Cottage, uncreamed | 86 | 17.0 | .3 | 2.7 | 90 | 175 | | .4 | 710 | 104 | 10 | .03 | .28 | .1 | |
| Swiss | 370 | 27.5 | 28.0 | 1.7 | 925 | 563 | | .9 | | | 1,140 | .01 | .40 | .1 | |
| Brick | 370 | 22.2 | 30.5 | 1.9 | 730 | 455 | | .9 | | | 1,240 | | .45 | .1 | |
| CHERRIES, sour, red, raw | 58 | 1.2 | .3 | 14.3 | 29 | 19 | 14 | .4 | 2 | 191 | 1,000 | .05 | .06 | .4 | 10 |
| sweet, raw | 70 | 1.3 | .3 | 17.4 | 22 | 19 | 9 | .4 | 2 | 191 | 110 | .05 | .06 | .4 | 10 |
| frozen, sour, red | 55 | 1.0 | .4 | 13.4 | 13 | 22 | 10 | .7 | 2 | 188 | 1,000 | .04 | .07 | .3 | 5 |
| CHESTNUTS, fresh | 194 | 2.9 | 1.5 | 42.1 | 27 | 88 | 41 | 1.7 | 6 | 454 | | .22 | .22 | .6 | |
| COCONUT MEAT, fresh | 346 | 3.5 | 35.3 | 9.4 | 13 | 95 | 46 | 1.7 | 23 | 256 | 0 | .05 | .02 | .5 | 3 |
| dried | 662 | 7.2 | 64.9 | 23.0 | 26 | 187 | 90 | 3.3 | | 588 | 0 | .06 | .04 | .6 | 0 |
| COCONUT WATER, from green coconuts | 22 | .3 | .2 | 4.7 | 20 | 13 | 28 | .3 | 25 | 147 | 0 | trace | trace | .1 | 2 |
| COLLARDS, raw, leaves | 45 | 4.8 | 0.8 | 7.5 | 250 | 82 | 57 | 1.5 | | 450 | 9,300 | 0.16 | .31 | 1.7 | 152 |
| cooked | 33 | 3.6 | .7 | 5.1 | 188 | 52 | 38 | .8 | | 262 | 7,800 | .11 | .20 | 1.2 | 76 |
| CORN, whole-grain, dried, raw | 348 | 8.9 | 3.9 | 72.0 | 22 | 268 | 147 | 2.1 | 1 | 284 | 490 | .37 | .12 | 2.2 | |
| SWEET, on-the-cob, raw | 96 | 3.5 | 1.0 | 22.0 | 3 | 111 | 48 | .7 | trace | 280 | 400 | .15 | .12 | 1.7 | 12 |
| cooked on the cob | 91 | 3.3 | 1.0 | 21.0 | 3 | 89 | 19 | .6 | trace | 196 | 400 | .12 | .10 | 1.4 | 9 |
| flour | 368 | 7.8 | 2.6 | 76.8 | 6 | 164 | 106 | 1.8 | | | 340 | .20 | .06 | 1.4 | |
| bread, whole-grain | 207 | 7.4 | 7.2 | 29.1 | 120 | 211 | | 1.1 | 628 | 157 | 150 | .13 | .19 | .6 | |
| CRANBERRIES, raw | 46 | .4 | .7 | 10.8 | 14 | 10 | 8 | .5 | 2 | 82 | 40 | .03 | .02 | .1 | 11 |
| CUCUMBERS, raw | 15 | .9 | .1 | 3.4 | 25 | 27 | 11 | 1.1 | 6 | 160 | 250 | .03 | .04 | .2 | 11 |

Nutritive values per 100 grams, edible portion.

| Food | Calories | Protein (g) | Fat (g) | Carbohydrate (g) | Calcium (mg) | Phosphorus (mg) | Magnesium (mg) | Iron (mg) | Sodium (mg) | Potassium (mg) | Vitamin A (IU) | Thiamine (mg) | Riboflavin (mg) | Niacin (mg) | Vitamin C (mg) |
|---|---|---|---|---|---|---|---|---|---|---|---|---|---|---|---|
| CURRANTS, black, raw | 54 | 1.7 | .1 | 13.1 | 60 | 40 | 15 | 1.1 | 3 | 372 | 230 | .05 | .05 | .3 | 200 |
| DANDELION GREENS, raw | 45 | 2.7 | .7 | 9.2 | 187 | 66 | 36 | 3.1 | 76 | 397 | 14,000 | .19 | .26 |  | 35 |
| DATES | 274 | 2.2 | .5 | 72.9 | 59 | 63 | 58 | 3.0 | 1 | 648 | 50 | .09 | .10 | 2.2 | 0 |
| EGGS, whole, raw | 163 | 12.9 | 11.5 | .9 | 54 | 205 | 11 | 2.3 | 122 | 129 | 1,180 | .11 | .30 | .1 | 0 |
| yolks, raw | 348 | 16.0 | 30.6 | .6 | 141 | 569 | 16 | 5.5 | 52 | 98 | 3,400 | .22 | .44 |  | 0 |
| cooked, whole | 163 | 12.9 | 11.5 | .9 | 54 | 205 |  | 2.3 | 122 | 29 | 1,180 | .09 | .28 | .1 | 0 |
| EGGPLANT, cooked | 19 | 1.0 | .2 | 4.1 | 11 | 21 | 10 | .6 | 1 | 50 | 10 | .05 | .04 | .5 | 3 |
| ELDERBERRIES, raw | 72 | 2.6 | .5 | 16.4 | 38 | 28 |  | 1.6 |  | 300 | 600 | .07 | .06 | .5 | 36 |
| ENDIVE, raw | 20 | 1.7 | .1 | 4.1 | 181 | 54 | 10 | 1.7 | 14 | 294 | 3,300 | .07 | .14 | .5 | 10 |
| FIGS, raw | 80 | 1.2 | .3 | 20.3 | 35 | 22 | 20 | .6 | 2 | 194 | 80 | .06 | .05 | .4 | 2 |
| dried | 274 | 4.3 | 1.3 | 69.1 | 126 | 77 | 71 | 3.0 | 34 | 640 | 80 | .10 | .10 | .7 | 0 |
| FILBERTS (hazelnuts) | 634 | 12.6 | 62.4 | 16.7 | 209 | 337 | 184 | 3.4 | 2 | 704 | trace | .46 |  | .9 | trace |
| GARLIC, raw | 137 | 6.2 | .2 | 30.8 | 29 | 202 | 36 | 1.5 | 19 | 529 | trace | .25 | .08 | .5 | 15 |
| GOOSEBERRIES, raw | 39 | 0.8 | .2 | 9.7 | 18 | 15 | 9 | 0.5 | 1 | 155 | 290 |  |  |  | 33 |
| GRAPEFRUIT, raw | 41 | .5 | .1 | 10.6 | 16 | 16 | 12 | .4 | 1 | 135 | 80 | .04 | .02 | .2 | 38 |
| juice | 39 | .5 | .1 | 9.2 | 9 | 15 | 12 | .2 |  | 162 | 80 | .04 | .02 | .2 | 38 |
| GRAPES, raw | 69 | 1.3 | 1.0 | 15.7 | 16 | 12 | 13 | .4 | 3 | 158 | 100 | .05 | .03 | .3 | 4 |
| juice, bottled | 66 | .2 | trace | 16.6 | 11 | 12 | 13 | .3 | 2 | 116 |  | .04 | .02 | .2 | trace |
| GUAVAS, whole, raw | 62 | .8 | .6 | 15. | 23 | 42 | 13 | .9 | 4 | 289 | 280 | .05 | .05 | 1.2 | 242 |
| HONEY | 304 | .3 | 0 | 82.3 | 5 | 6 | 3 | .5 | 5 | 51 | 0 | trace | .04 | .3 | 1 |
| HORSERADISH, raw | 87 | 3.2 | .3 | 19.7 | 140 | 64 | 34 | 1.4 | 8 | 564 |  | .07 |  |  | 81 |
| KALE, leaves, raw | 53 | 6.0 | .8 | 9.0 | 249 | 93 | 37 | 2.7 | 75 | 378 | 10,000 | .17 | .26 | 2.1 | 186 |
| cooked | 39 | 4.5 | .7 | 6.1 | 187 | 58 | 37 | 1.6 | 43 | 221 | 8,300 | .10 | .18 | 1.6 | 93 |
| KELP, raw |  | 5.0 | 1.1 |  | 1,093 | 240 | 740 | 3.7 | 3,007 | 5,273 |  |  |  |  | 5-140 |
| KOHLRABI, raw | 29 | 2.0 | .1 | 6.6 | 41 | 51 | 37 | .5 | 8 | 372 | 20 | .06 | .04 | .3 | 66 |
| KUMQUATS, raw | 65 | .9 | .1 | 17.1 | 63 | 23 |  | .4 | 7 | 236 | 600 | .08 | .10 |  | 36 |
| LEMONS, peeled, raw | 27 | 1.1 | .3 | 8.2 | 26 | 16 | 10 | .6 | 2 | 138 | 20 | .04 | .02 | .1 | 53 |
| LEMON JUICE, raw | 25 | .5 | .2 | 8.0 | 7 | 10 | 8 | .2 | 1 | 141 | 20 | .03 | .01 | .1 | 46 |
| LENTILS, dry, cooked | 106 | 7.8 | trace | 19.3 | 25 | 119 | 80 | 2.1 |  | 249 | 20 | .07 | .06 | .6 | 0 |
| LETTUCE, raw, romaine | 18 | 1.3 | .3 | 3.5 | 68 | 25 |  | 1.4 | 9 | 264 | 1,900 | .05 | .08 | .4 | 18 |
| iceberg, New York | 13 | .9 | .1 | 2.9 | 20 | 22 | 11 | .5 | 9 | 175 | 330 | .06 | .06 | .3 | 6 |
| MANGOS, raw | 66 | .7 | .4 | 16.8 | 10 | 13 | 18 | .4 | 7 | 189 | 4,800 | .05 | .05 | 1.1 | 35 |

| FOOD | CALORIES | PROTEINS grams | FATS grams | CARBOHYDRATES grams | CALCIUM mg. | PHOSPHORUS mg. | MAGNESIUM mg. | IRON mg. | SODIUM mg. | POTASSIUM mg. | VITAMIN A VALUE IU | B₁ mg. | B₂ mg. | NIACIN mg. | VITAMIN C mg. |
|---|---|---|---|---|---|---|---|---|---|---|---|---|---|---|---|
| MILK, cow's, whole | 65 | 3.5 | 3.5 | 4.9 | 118 | 93 | 13 | trace | 50 | 144 | 140 | .03 | .17 | .1 | 1 |
| skim | 36 | 3.6 | .1 | 5.1 | 121 | 95 | 14 | trace | 52 | 145 | trace | .04 | .18 | .1 | 1 |
| dry, whole | 502 | 26.4 | 27.5 | 38.2 | 909 | 708 | 98 | .5 | 405 | 1,330 | 1,130 | .29 | 1.46 | .7 | 6 |
| dry, skim non-instant | 363 | 35.9 | .8 | 52.3 | 1,308 | 1,016 | 143 | .6 | 532 | 1,745 | 30 | .35 | 1.80 | .9 | 7 |
| MILK, goat's, raw | 67 | 3.2 | 4.0 | 4.6 | 129 | 106 | 17 | .1 | 34 | 180 | 160 | .04 | .11 | .3 | 1 |
| MILLET, whole-grain | 327 | 9.9 | 2.9 | 72.9 | 20 | 311 | 162 | 6.8 | — | 430 | 0 | .73 | .38 | 2.3 | 0 |
| MOLASSES, blackstrap | 213 | — | — | 55 | 684 | 84 | 258 | 16.1 | 96 | 2,927 | — | .11 | .19 | 2.0 | — |
| MUSHROOMS, cultivated, raw | 28 | 2.7 | .3 | 4.4 | 6 | 116 | 13 | .8 | 15 | 414 | trace | .10 | .46 | 4.2 | 3 |
| MUSKMELONS, raw, cantaloupe | 30 | .7 | .1 | 7.5 | 14 | 16 | 16 | .4 | 12 | 251 | 3,400 | .04 | .03 | .6 | 33 |
| honeydew | 33 | .8 | .3 | 7.7 | 14 | 16 | — | .4 | 12 | 251 | 40 | .04 | .03 | .6 | 23 |
| MUSTARD GREENS, raw | 31 | 3.0 | .5 | 5.6 | 183 | 50 | 27 | 3.0 | 32 | 377 | 7,000 | .11 | .22 | .8 | 97 |
| NECTARINES, raw | 64 | .6 | trace | 17.1 | 4 | 24 | 13 | .5 | 6 | 294 | 1,650 | — | — | — | 13 |
| OATMEAL or rolled oats, dry | 390 | 14.2 | 7.2 | 68.2 | 53 | 405 | 144 | 4.5 | 2 | 352 | 0 | .60 | .14 | 1.0 | 0 |
| cooked | 55 | 2.0 | 1.0 | 9.7 | 9 | 57 | 21 | .6 | — | 61 | 0 | .08 | .02 | .1 | 0 |
| OKRA, raw | 36 | 2.4 | .3 | 7.6 | 92 | 51 | 41 | .6 | 3 | 249 | 520 | .17 | .21 | 1.0 | 31 |
| ONIONS, mature, raw | 38 | 1.5 | .1 | 8.7 | 27 | 36 | 12 | .5 | 10 | 157 | 40 | .03 | .04 | .2 | 10 |
| green, bulb & top | 36 | 1.5 | .2 | 8.2 | 51 | 39 | — | 1.0 | 5 | 237 | 2,000 | .05 | .05 | .4 | 32 |
| ORANGES, peeled, raw | 49 | 1.0 | .2 | 12.2 | 41 | 20 | 11 | .4 | 1 | 200 | 200 | .10 | .04 | .4 | 50 |
| ORANGE JUICE, raw | 45 | .7 | .2 | 10.2 | 11 | 17 | 11 | .2 | 1 | 200 | 200 | .09 | .03 | .4 | 50 |
| PAPAYA, raw | 39 | .6 | .1 | 10.0 | 20 | 16 | — | .3 | 3 | 234 | 1,750 | .04 | .04 | .3 | 56 |
| PARSLEY, raw | 44 | 3.6 | .6 | 8.5 | 203 | 63 | 41 | 6.2 | 45 | 727 | 8,500 | .12 | .26 | 1.2 | 172 |
| PARSNIPS, raw | 76 | 1.7 | .5 | 17.5 | 50 | 77 | 32 | .7 | 12 | 541 | 30 | .07 | .08 | .1 | 10 |
| PEACHES, raw | 38 | .6 | .1 | 9.7 | 9 | 19 | 10 | .5 | 1 | 202 | 1,330 | .02 | .05 | .1 | 7 |
| PEANUTS, raw, with skins | 564 | 26.0 | 47.5 | 18.6 | 69 | 401 | 206 | 2.1 | 5 | 674 | — | 1.14 | .13 | 17.2 | 0 |

164

| | | | | | | | | | | | | | | | |
|---|---|---|---|---|---|---|---|---|---|---|---|---|---|---|---|
| PEARS, raw | 61 | .7 | .4 | 15.3 | 8 | 11 | 7 | 130 | .3 | 2 | 20 | .02 | .04 | .1 | 4 |
| PEAS, raw, from pods | 53 | 3.4 | .2 | 12.0 | 62 | 90 | 35 | 170 | .7 | | 680 | .28 | .12 | | 21 |
| green, cooked | 71 | 5.4 | .4 | 12.1 | 23 | 99 | | 196 | 1.8 | 1 | 540 | .28 | .11 | 2.3 | 20 |
| split, cooked | 115 | 8.0 | .3 | 20.8 | 11 | 89 | | 296 | 1.7 | | 40 | .15 | .09 | .9 | |
| PECANS | 687 | 9.2 | 71.2 | 14.6 | 73 | 289 | 142 | 603 | 2.4 | trace | 130 | .86 | .13 | .9 | 2 |
| PEPPERS, raw, sweet, green | 22 | 1.2 | .2 | 4.8 | 9 | 22 | 18 | 213 | .7 | | 420 | .08 | .08 | .5 | 128 |
| raw, red | 31 | 1.4 | .3 | 7.1 | 13 | 30 | | 310 | .6 | | 4,450 | .08 | .08 | .5 | 204 |
| PERSIMMONS, raw | 127 | .8 | .4 | 33.5 | 27 | 26 | 8 | 146 | 2.5 | 1 | | | | | 66 |
| PINEAPPLE, raw | 52 | 0.4 | 0.2 | 13.7 | 17 | 8 | 13 | 149 | 0.5 | 1 | 70 | .09 | .03 | .2 | 17 |
| juice, canned, unsweetened | 55 | .4 | .1 | 13.5 | 15 | 9 | 12 | 170 | .3 | 1 | 50 | .05 | .02 | .2 | 9 |
| PLUMS, prune-type, raw | 75 | .8 | .2 | 19.7 | 12 | 18 | 9 | 170 | .5 | 1 | 300 | .03 | .03 | .5 | 4 |
| POTATOES, raw | 76 | 2.1 | .1 | 17.1 | 7 | 53 | 34 | 407 | .6 | 3 | trace | .10 | .04 | 1.5 | 20 |
| baked in skin | 93 | 2.6 | .1 | 21.1 | 9 | 65 | | 503 | .7 | 4 | trace | .10 | .04 | 1.7 | 20 |
| boiled in skin | 76 | 2.1 | .1 | 17.1 | 7 | 53 | 12 | 407 | .6 | 3 | trace | .09 | .04 | 1.5 | 16 |
| PUMPKIN, raw | 26 | 1.0 | .1 | 6.5 | 21 | 44 | | 340 | .8 | 1 | 1,600 | .05 | .11 | .6 | 9 |
| PUMPKIN SEEDS, dry | 553 | 29.0 | 46.7 | 15.0 | 51 | 1,144 | 15 | | 11.2 | | 70 | .24 | .19 | 2.4 | |
| RADISHES, raw | 17 | 1.0 | .1 | 3.6 | 30 | 31 | 35 | 322 | 1.0 | 18 | 10 | .03 | .03 | .3 | 26 |
| RAISINS, natural, uncooked | 289 | 2.5 | .2 | 77.4 | 62 | 101 | 30 | 763 | 3.5 | 27 | 20 | .11 | .08 | .5 | 1 |
| RASPBERRIES, raw, black | 73 | 1.5 | 1.4 | 15.7 | 30 | 22 | 20 | 199 | .9 | 1 | trace | .03 | .09 | .9 | 18 |
| red | 57 | 1.2 | .5 | 13.6 | 22 | 22 | 29 | 168 | .9 | | 130 | .03 | .09 | .9 | 25 |
| RICE, brown, cooked | 119 | 2.5 | .6 | 25.5 | 12 | 73 | | 70 | .5 | 3 | 0 | .09 | .02 | 1.4 | 0 |
| RICE BRAN | 276 | 13.3 | 15.8 | 50.8 | 76 | 1,386 | | 1,495 | 19.4 | trace | 0 | 2.26 | .25 | 29.8 | 0 |
| RICE POLISHINGS | 265 | 12.1 | 12.8 | 57.7 | 69 | 1,106 | 115 | 714 | 16.1 | trace | 0 | 1.84 | .18 | 28.2 | 0 |
| RUTABAGAS, raw | 46 | 1.1 | .1 | 11.0 | 66 | 39 | 73 | 239 | .4 | 5 | 580 | .07 | .07 | 1.1 | 43 |
| cooked | 35 | .9 | .1 | 8.2 | 59 | 31 | | 167 | .3 | 4 | 550 | .06 | .06 | .8 | 26 |
| RYE, whole-grain | 334 | 12.1 | 1.7 | 73.4 | 38 | 376 | 181 | 467 | 3.7 | 1 | 0 | .43 | .22 | 1.6 | 0 |
| flour, dark | 327 | 16.3 | 2.6 | 68.1 | 54 | 536 | 265 | 360 | 4.5 | 1 | 0 | .61 | .22 | 2.7 | 0 |
| SAUERKRAUT, solids and liquid | 18 | 1.0 | .2 | 4.0 | 36 | 18 | | 140 | .5 | | 50 | .03 | .04 | .2 | 14 |
| SESAME SEEDS, dry, whole | 563 | 18.6 | 49.1 | 21.6 | 1,160 | 616 | | 725 | 10.5 | 60 | 30 | .98 | .24 | 5.4 | 0 |
| SOYBEANS, dry, raw | 403 | 34.1 | 17.7 | 33.5 | 226 | 554 | | 1,677 | 8.4 | 5 | 80 | 1.10 | .31 | 2.2 | |
| cooked | 130 | 11.0 | 5.7 | 10.8 | 73 | 179 | | 540 | 2.7 | 2 | 30 | .21 | .09 | .6 | 0 |
| sprouted, raw | 46 | 6.2 | 1.4 | 5.3 | 48 | 67 | | | 1.0 | | 80 | .23 | .20 | .8 | 13 |
| sprouted, cooked | 38 | 5.3 | 1.4 | 3.7 | 43 | 50 | | | .7 | | 80 | .16 | .15 | .7 | 4 |

|  | | | | | | | | | | | | | | |
|---|---|---|---|---|---|---|---|---|---|---|---|---|---|---|
| SOYBEAN CURD (TOFU) | 72 | 7.8 | 4.2 | 2.4 | 128 | 126 | 111 | 1.9 | 7 | 42 | 0 | .06 | .03 | .1 |
| SOYBEAN FLOUR, full-fat | 421 | 36.7 | 20.3 | 30.4 | 199 | 558 | 247 | 8.4 | 1 | 1,660 | 110 | .85 | .31 | 2.1 |
| SOYBEAN MILK, powder | 429 | 41.8 | 20.3 | 28.0 | 278 | — | 300 | — | — | — | — | — | — | — |
| SPINACH, raw | 26 | 3.2 | .3 | 4.3 | 93 | 51 | 88 | 3.1 | 71 | 470 | 8,100 | .10 | .20 | .6 |
| cooked | 23 | 3.0 | .3 | 3.6 | 93 | 38 | 65 | 2.2 | 50 | 324 | 8,000 | .07 | .14 | .5 |
| SQUASH, summer, all varieties, raw | 19 | 1.1 | 1.1 | 4.2 | 28 | 29 | 16 | 0.4 | 1 | 202 | 410 | .05 | .09 | 1.0 |
| cooked | 14 | .9 | .1 | 3.1 | 25 | 25 | 16 | 0.4 | 1 | 141 | 370 | .05 | .08 | .8 |
| winter, raw | 50 | 1.4 | .3 | 12.4 | 22 | 38 | 17 | .6 | 1 | 369 | 3,700 | .05 | .11 | .6 |
| cooked (baked) | 63 | 1.8 | .4 | 15.4 | 28 | 48 | 17 | .8 | 1 | 461 | 4,200 | .05 | .13 | .7 |
| STRAWBERRIES, raw | 37 | .7 | .5 | 8.4 | 21 | 21 | 12 | 1.0 | 1 | 164 | 60 | .03 | .07 | .6 |
| SUNFLOWER SEED KERNELS, dry | 560 | 24.0 | 47.3 | 19.9 | 120 | 837 | 38 | 7.1 | 30 | 920 | 50 | 1.96 | .23 | 5.4 |
| TOMATOES, ripe, raw | 22 | 1.1 | .2 | 4.7 | 13 | 27 | 14 | .5 | 3 | 244 | 900 | .06 | .04 | .7 |
| TOMATO JUICE, canned | 19 | .9 | .1 | 4.3 | 7 | 18 | 10 | .9 | 200 | 227 | 800 | .05 | .03 | .8 |
| TURNIPS, raw | 30 | 1.0 | .2 | 6.6 | 39 | 30 | 20 | .5 | 49 | 268 | trace | .04 | .07 | .6 |
| cooked | 23 | .8 | .2 | 4.9 | 35 | 24 | — | .4 | 34 | 188 | trace | .04 | .05 | .3 |
| TURNIP GREENS, raw | 28 | 3.0 | .3 | 5.0 | 246 | 58 | 58 | 1.8 | — | — | 7,600 | .21 | .39 | .8 |
| WALNUTS, black | 628 | 20.5 | 59.3 | 14.8 | trace | 570 | 190 | 6.0 | 3 | 460 | 300 | .22 | .11 | .7 |
| English | 651 | 14.8 | 64.0 | 15.8 | 99 | 380 | 131 | 3.1 | 2 | 450 | 30 | .33 | .13 | .9 |
| WATERCRESS, raw | 19 | 2.2 | .3 | 3.0 | 151 | 54 | 20 | 1.7 | 52 | 282 | 4,900 | .08 | .16 | .9 |
| WATERMELON, raw | 26 | .5 | .2 | 6.4 | 7 | 10 | 8 | .5 | 1 | 100 | 590 | .03 | .03 | .2 |
| WHEAT, whole-grain, spring | 330 | 14.0 | 2.2 | 69.1 | 36 | 383 | 160 | 3.1 | 3 | 370 | — | .57 | .12 | 4.3 |
| winter | 330 | 12.3 | 1.8 | 71.7 | 46 | 354 | 160 | 3.4 | 3 | 370 | — | .52 | .12 | 4.3 |
| WHEAT BRAN | 213 | 16.0 | 4.6 | 61.9 | 119 | 1,276 | 490 | 14.9 | 9 | 1,121 | 0 | .72 | .35 | 21.0 |
| WHEAT GERM, raw | 363 | 26.6 | 10.9 | 46.7 | 72 | 1,118 | 336 | 9.4 | 3 | 827 | 0 | 2.01 | .68 | 4.2 |
| WHEY, powder | 349 | 12.9 | 1.1 | 73.5 | 646 | 589 | 130 | 1.4 | — | — | 50 | .50 | 2.51 | .8 |
| YAM, tuber, raw | 101 | 2.1 | .2 | 23.2 | 20 | 69 | 31 | .6 | — | 600 | — | .10 | .04 | .5 |
| YEAST, brewer's debittered | 283 | 38.8 | 1.0 | 38.4 | 210 | 1,753 | 231 | 17.3 | 121 | 1,894 | trace | 15.61 | 4.28 | 37.9 |
| torula | 277 | 38.6 | 1.0 | 37.0 | 424 | 1,713 | 165 | 19.3 | 15 | 2,046 | trace | 14.01 | 5.06 | 44.4 |
| YOGURT, from whole milk | 62 | 3.0 | 3.4 | 4.9 | 111 | 87 | 12 | trace | 47 | 132 | 140 | .03 | .16 | .1 |
| from skimmed milk | 50 | 3.4 | 1.7 | 5.2 | 120 | 94 | 13 | trace | 51 | 143 | 70 | .04 | .18 | .1 |

SOURCES: Agriculture Handbook No. 8., U.S. Dept. Agric. Washington, D.C.; Home and Garden Bulletin No. 72.

# Glossary

Absorption    the process whereby nutrients pass through the intestines into the blood stream.

Acid    any water soluble sour compound containing hydrogen, which will react with a base to form a salt.

Alkaloids    bitter organic bases containing nitrogen, found in seed plants.

Allergy    an exaggerated response by the body (sneezing, itching, skin rashes, etc.) to certain irritating substances.

Amino acids    a group of organic nitrogen containing compounds necessary for the building of protein molecules.

Anemia    a deficiency of red blood cells, hemoglobin, or total blood volume.

Anion    an ion carrying a negative charge

Antagonist    a drug that neutralizes the action of another drug.

Antibiotic    a substance produced by a microorganism which is capable of destroying other microorganisms.

Antibody    a substance in the blood that produces immunity to a specific virus or bacteria.

Anticoagulant    a substance that prevents or hinders blood clotting.

Antihistamine    a medication used for treating allergic reactions by inactivating histamines.

Antioxidant — a substance which prevents oxidation or inhibits reactions promoted by the presence of oxygen.

Arteriosclerosis — thickening, hardening, or loss of elasticity of the walls of blood vessels and arteries.

Assimilate — to absorb nutrients into the body.

Atherosclerosis — hardening of the arteries due to deposits of fatty substances on the inner lining of the arteries. A form of arteriosclerosis.

Bacteria — single celled microscopic organisms that are beneficial or harmful to the body.

Base — water soluble bitter compound capable of neutralizing an acid to form a salt.

Biological — relating to life and living processes.

Calcification — the deposit of calcium in body tissues.

Capillary — the smallest vessels of the blood system connecting arterioles with venules.

Carbohydrates — neutral compounds of carbon, hydrogen, and oxygen such as sugars, starches, and celluloses, which are formed by green plants.

Carcinogen — a substance which produces cancer.

Carotene — orange or red pigments produced by plants which can be converted into vitamin A by the body.

Carpal tunnel syndrome — pain, tenderness, and weakness of the muscles of the thumb caused by pressure on the median nerve at the point at which it goes through the carpal tunnel of the wrist.

| | |
|---|---|
| Catabolism | the breakdown of complex compounds during metabolism with a release of energy. |
| Catalyst | a substance that stimulates and speeds up a chemical reaction. |
| Cation | an ion carrying a positive charge. |
| Cellulose | a complex, nondigestible carbohydrate found in the cell walls of plants. |
| Cement, inter-cellular | a substance found between the cells, which holds them together. |
| Central nervous system | the nervous system containing the brain, spinal cord, and the nerves branching out from the spinal cord. |
| Cholesterol | a steriod found in bile, gall stones, fats, blood, and brain tissue. |
| Chronic | of long duration, or frequent recurrence; not acute. |
| Circulatory system | transportation of blood through the arteries and veins. |
| Cirrhosis | fibrosis of the liver, replacement of liver cells by fibrous tissue, and obstruction of blood flow through the liver. |
| Coagulation | the formation of a blood clot. |
| Coenzyme | a non-protein compound, usually a vitamin or mineral, which forms the active portion of an enzyme system. |
| Collagen | the main constituent of connective tissue and bones; yields gelatin or glue when heated. |
| Conjunctivitis | inflammation of the conjunctiva, the membrane covering the inside of the eyelid and part of the eyeball. |

| | |
|---|---|
| Contraceptive | drug or device to prevent conception, or pregnancy. |
| Deficiency | a lack of vitamins or minerals necessary for good health. |
| Degeneration | deterioration of tissues or organs, with a loss of vitality and function, leading to destruction of cells. |
| Dermatitis | inflammation of the skin. |
| Detoxify | remove the poisonous properties from a substance. |
| Disorder | a disturbance of normal physical or mental functions. |
| Diuretic | an agent that increases the flow of urine. |
| DNA | deoxyribonucleic acid, the nucleic acid present in the chromosomes and containing the hereditary characteristics. |
| Eczema | inflammation of the skin characterized by redness, itching, and oozing vesicles which form crusts and scales. |
| Edema | excess accumulation of fluid in cells, tissues, or serous cavities, resulting in swelling. |
| Electrolyte | a substance such as sodium, potassium, or chloride, which conducts an electrical current when in solution. |
| Enzyme | a protein which acts as a catalyst to stimulate chemical changes in other substances without being changed itself. |
| Epithelial tissue | membranes that line all the hollow organs of the digestive, urinary, and respiratory systems, and also the skin. |

| | |
|---|---|
| Extracellular | occuring outside the cells. |
| Fats | greasy or oily substances found in animal tissues and many plants, glycerides of fatty acids; a major source of energy. |
| Fat-soluble vitamins | those vitamins that must be dissolved in dietary fats, or need bile salts in order to be absorbed (A, D, E, and K). |
| Fatty acids | an acid originating from the hydrolysis of fats, such as oleic, stearic, or palmitic acid. |
| Fermentation | a chemical breakdown in an organic substance by the action of enzymes to produce simple compounds. |
| Gastrointestinal | relating to the stomach and intestines. |
| Gingivitis | inflammation of the gums. |
| Glaucoma | an eye disease characterized by increased pressure within the eyeball and gradual loss of sight. |
| Glucose | the simple sugar formed by the complete breakdown of complex carbohydrates, which is assimilated by the body. |
| Glycogen | the form in which carbohydrates are stored in the liver. |
| Glycosuria | the presence of sugar in the urine. |
| Goiter | enlarged thyroid gland. |
| Goitrogen | any substance that produces goiter. |
| Hemoglobin | the iron-containing pigment in the red blood cells which carries oxygen to the cells. |
| Hemorrhage | profuse bleeding, internal or external. |

| | |
|---|---|
| Histamine | a substance which causes dilation and increased permeability of the blood vessels in allergic reactions. |
| Hormone | a chemical substance secreted into the blood stream by one organ which affects the function of another organ. |
| Hydrochloric acid | an acid secreted by the lining of the stomach; is helpful in digestion. |
| Hypoglycemia | abnormally low level of sugar in the blood. |
| Hypoxia | deficiency of oxygen in the tissues and blood. |
| Infection | state produced by growth of harmful bacteria, viruses, or parasites in the body. |
| Inflammation | a local response to cellular injury as a result of trauma or disease; marked by redness, pain, heat, and swelling. |
| Inorganic | not organic or related to living organisms; compounds not containing carbon. |
| Insulin | a pancreatic hormone secreted by the islets of Langerhans which regulates the metabolism of carbohydrates. |
| Intercellular | between the cells. |
| Intestinal flora | bacteria normally present in the intestines. |
| Intracellular | within the cells. |
| Intravenous | within the vein. |
| Lactation | secretion of milk in mammals. |

| | |
|---|---|
| Legumes | the fruit or pod of beans, peas, lentils, etc. |
| Lipids | fats and fat-like substances. |
| Malabsorption | abnormal or inadequate gastrointestinal absorption. |
| Malnutrition | faulty or inadequate nutrition. |
| Megavitamin | very large doses of vitamins used for therapeutic purposes. |
| Metabolism | the chemical processes consisting of anabolism, or energy consumption, where small molecules are converted into large ones; and catabolism, or energy production, whereby large molecules are broken down into small molecules. |
| Mineral | an inorganic substance which does not contain carbon. |
| Mitochondria | slender microscopic filaments or rods found in cells, which are the source of energy in the cell; also involved in protein synthesis and lipid metabolism. |
| Molecule | the smallest quantity of a substance which retains all its chemical properties. |
| Naturopath | a practitioner who treats disease using natural remedies such as foods, herbs, water, etc. |
| Nucleic acids | substances found in the chromosomes, the carriers of hereditary material. |
| Nucleoproteins | the combination of one of the proteins with nucleic acid to form a conjugated protein found in the cell nuclei. |

Nutrient            any item of food that provides nourish-
                    ment.

Organic             of plant or animal origin; containing
                    carbon.

Oxalic acid         a poisonous acid found in various plants
                    as oxalates.

Oxidation           the process of combining with oxygen.

Oxygenation         the process of supplying oxygen.

Pathogenic          capable of causing disease.

Pernicious          severe; usually fatal.

Phospholipid        a fat containing phosphorus; lecithin,
                    phosphatidic acids, sphingomyelin, etc.

Placebo             an inactive substance given in place of a
                    medication or drug to satisfy the patient
                    or used as a control in experiments.

Platelets           small flattened disks in the blood which
                    are involved in blood clotting.

Pollen              microspores in flowering plants which
                    are carried by insects and winds and may
                    cause allergies.

Preservatives       additives used to prevent spoilage.

Prophylactic        preventive.

Protein             combinations of amino acids found in all
                    cells and involved in all essential
                    functions of the body.

Psoriasis

a chronic skin disease characterized by reddish patches covered with silvery scales, occurring on elbows, knees, chest, and scalp.

Respiratory system

organs involved in breathing — the nose, pharynx, larynx, bronchial tubes, and lungs.

RNA

ribonucleic acid; a nucleic acid found in all cells; responsible for the transmission of hereditary information.

Seborrhea

a skin disease characterized by over-secretion of the sebaceous glands.

Schizophrenia

a psychosis characterized by withdrawal from reality.

Supplement

nutrients taken in addition to the regular diet to complete the amount of vitamins and minerals needed by the body.

Symptom

indication of disease.

Syndrome

a group of signs and symptoms which occur together and constitute a particular disease.

Synergist

an agent involved in the process of synergism, whereby two agents such as drugs, organs, or muscles, working in cooperation, produce an effect which neither could produce alone, or which is greater than the total effect produced by each agent working alone.

Synthesis            the process of building up; the formation
                     of complex compounds from simpler
                     compounds.

Synthetic            produced artificially.

Tannin               an astringent substance found in many
                     plants and used in tanning, dyeing, and
                     for medicinal purposes.

Therapeutic          relating to the treatment of disease.

Thrombo-             inflammation of a vein with the formation
   phlebitis         of a blood clot.

Tissue               a group of similar cells and the inter-
                     cellular substances around them which
                     form the structural materials of the body.

Toxicity             poisonous effects.

Toxin                poisonous substance.

Transamination       transfer of an amino group from an
                     alpha-amino acid to an alpha-keto acid.

Vasodilator          an agent that causes dilation of the blood
                     vessels.

Vitamin              organic substances found in food in
                     minute quantities which are essential for
                     normal metabolism.

Water soluble        vitamin C and the B-complex vita-
   vitamins          mins; those which dissolve in water.

# Bibliography

Adams, Catherine F., *Nutritive Value of American Foods in Common Units,* Agriculture Handbook No. 456, Washington D.C.: U.S. Department of Agriculture, 1975.

Airola, Paavo, *The Airola Diet & Cookbook,* Phoenix, AZ: Health Plus Publishers, 1981.

Airola, Paavo, *Everywoman's Book,* Phoenix, AZ: Health Plus Publishers, 1979.

Airola, Paavo, *How To Get Well,* Phoenix, AZ: Health Plus Publishers, 1974.

Alhadeff, Leslie, C. T. Gualtieri, M. Lipton, "Toxic Effects of Water-Soluble Vitamins," *Nutrition Review,* 42:2, February, 1984.

Benowicz, Robert J., *Vitamins & You,* New York, NY: Grosset & Dunlap, 1979.

Berkow, Robert (ed.), *The Merck Manual,* 13th ed., Rahway, NJ: Merck & Co., Inc., 1977.

Bowen, H.J.M., and A. Peggs, "Determination of the Silicon Content of Food," *Journal of Sci Food Agric.,* 1984, 35:1225-1229.

Cook, J.D., and E.R. Monsen, "Vitamin C, The Common Cold and Iron Absorption," *American Journal of Clinical Nutrition,* 30:235-241, 1977.

Darby, W.J., K.W. McNutt, and E.N. Todhunter, "Niacin," *Nutrition Review,* 33:289-297, 1975.

Donald, E.A., "The Vitamin $B_6$ Requirements of Young Women," pp. 226-237, *Human Vitamin $B_6$ Requirements,* National Academy of Sciences, Washington, D.C., 1978.

Doyle, Rodger P., and J.L. Redding, *The Complete Food Handbook,* New York, NY: Grove Press, Inc., 1979.

Ellenboger, Leon, *Controversies in Nutrition,* New York, NY: Churchill Livingston, Inc., 1981.

Faelten, Sharon, *Vitamins For Better Health,* Emmaus, PA: Rodale Press, 1982.

FAO/WHO (Food and Agriculture Organization/World Health Organization), "Requirements of Vitamin A, Thiamin, Riboflavin, and Niacin," Report of a joint FAO/WHO Expert Committee. FAO Nutrition Meeting Report Series No. 41, WHO Tech. Report, Series No. 362, WHO Geneva, 86 pp., 1967.

FAO/WHO, "Requirements of Ascorbic Acid, Vitamin D, Vitamin $B_{12}$, Folate, and Iron," World Health Organization Tech. Report Series No. 452, Geneva, Switzerland, 75 pp.

Food and Nutrition Board, *Recommended Dietary Allowances,* 9th revised edition, National Research Council, National Academy of Sciences, Washington, D.C., 1980.

FNB (Food and Nutrition Board, National Research Council), 1970. "Zinc in Human Nutrition," Proceedings of workshop, National Academy of Sciences, Washington, D.C., 50 pp., 1970.

Goodhart, Robert S. and Maurice E. Shils, *Modern Nutrition in Health and Disease,* 6th ed., Philadelphia, PA: Lea and Feibiger, 1980.

Human Nutrition Information Service, *Composition of Foods,* Agriculture Handbook No. 8 (1-12), Washington, D.C.: U.S. Department of Agriculture, 1984.

Linkswiler, H.M., "Vitamin $B_6$ Requirements of Men," pp. 279-290, *Human Vitamin $B_6$ Requirements,* National Academy of Sciences, Washington, D.C., 1978.

Marsh, A.C., and P.C. Koons, "The Sodium and Potassium Content of Selected Vegetables," *Journal of the American Dietetic Association,* 83:24, 1983.

McLaughlin, P.J., and John L. Weihrauch, "Vitamin E Content of Foods," *Journal of American Dietetic Association,* 175:647, December, 1979.

Morton, R.A. (ed.), *Fat Soluble Vitamins,* Pergamon Press, 1970.

Monsen, E.R., et al, "Estimation of Available Dietary Iron," *American Journal of Clinical Nutrition,* 31:134-141.

Natow, Annette, and JoAnn Heslin, *Nutrition for the Prime of Your Life,* New York, NY: McGraw Hill Book Company, 1983.

Nutrition Search, Inc., *Nutrition Almanac,* New York, NY: McGraw-Hill Book Company, 1979.

Orr, Martha Louise, *Pantothenic Acid, Vitamin $B_6$ and Vitamin $B_{12}$,* Home Economics Research Report No. 36, Washington, D.C.: U.S. Dept. of Agriculture, 1969.

Palmer, I.S., et al, "Selenium Intake and Urinary Excretion in Persons Living Near a High Selenium Area," *Journal of the American Dietetic Association,* 82:511, 1983.

Pennington, Jean, and Helen Nichols Church, *Food Values of Portions Commonly Used,* 13th ed., Philadelphia, PA: J.B. Lippincott, Co., 1980.

Prasad, A.S., "Deficiency of Zinc in Man and Its Toxicity," pp. 1-20, A.S. Prasad (ed.) *Trace Elements in Human Health and Diseases*, New York, NY: Academic Press, 1976.

Reilly, Conor, *Metal Contamination of Food*, Essex, England: Applied Science Publishers, Ltd., 1980.

Shilotri, P.G. and K.S. Bhat, "Effect of Mega Doses of Vitamin C on Bactericidal Activity of Leukocytes, *American Journal of Clinical Nutrition*, 30:1077-1081.

Shute, Evan, *The Heart and Vitamin E*, London, Canada: Evan Shute Foundation, 1963.

Shute, Wilfred E. and Harold Taub, *Vitamin E for Ailing and Healthy Hearts*, New York, NY: Pyramid House, 1969.

Spencer, H.L., et al, "Effect of a High Protein (meat) Intake on Calcium Metabolism in Man," *American Journal of Clinical Nutrition*, 31:2167-2180.

Sutker, L.R., and J.A. Driskell, "Vitamin E Status of Adolescent Girls," *Journal of the American Dietetic Association*, 83:678, 1983.

Taber, Clarence Wilbur, *Taber's Cyclopedic Medical Dictionary*, Philadelphia, PA: S.A. Davis Co., 9th ed., 1963.

Tobias, Alice L., Patricia J. Thompson, *Issues in Nutrition for the 1980's*, Monterey, CA: Wadsworth Health Sciences Division, 1980.

Tucherman, Murray M. and Salvatore J. Turco, *Human Nutrition*, Philadelphia, PA: Lea and Febiger, 1983.

Tuman, R.W., and Doisy, R.J., "The Role of Trace Elements in Human Nutrition and Metabolism," *Sourcebook of Food and Nutrition*, 2nd ed., Chicago, IL: Marquis Academic Media, 1980.

Underwood, Eric J., "Trace Element Imbalances of Interest to the Dietitian," *Journal of the American Dietetic Association*, February, 1978, pp. 177-179.

Underwood, E.J., *Trace Elements in Human and Animal Nutrition*, 4th ed., New York, NY: Academic Press, 1977.

Wacker, W.E.C., and A.F. Parisi, "Magnesium Metabolism," *New England Journal of Medicine*, 278:658-776.

WHO (World Health Organization) "Fluoride and Human Health," WHO Monograph Series No. 59, WHO, Geneva, 1970.

Wilkinson, R., "Absorption of Calcium, Phosphorus and Magnesium," pp. 36-112, B.E.C. Nordin (ed.) *Calcium, Phosphate and Magnesium Metabolism*, New York, NY: Churchill Livingston, Inc., 1976.

# INDEX

# W

# Z